Molar Pregnancy

What is a molar pregnancy or hydatidiform mole? Symptoms, causes and treatments.

Includes practical advice on recovery and preparing for future pregnancy.

By

Claudia Gordon

Published by Adhurst Publishing Ltd. 2014

Contents

Foreword

If you are reading this, then it is possible that you've either been diagnosed with a molar pregnancy yourself and are being treated for it or you know someone who is. Hopefully, this is comprehensive enough that it offers you some understanding of molar pregnancy as well as some of the complications that can arise from it. Losing a pregnancy can be devastating but it can be particularly challenging when a woman's health may continue to be at risk even after the pregnancy has ended and that is exactly what happens in both partial and complete molar pregnancies.

Unfortunately, despite the fact that thousands of women continue to live with complications from molar pregnancies every year, it is a health condition that not many people know about. Even some doctors seem to have little understanding of them, especially when it comes to the emotional impact that a woman can suffer from such a loss.

At the current time there is no way to prevent molar pregnancies from happening. Hopefully, however, with more education and research and by raising awareness there *will* be a way to prevent them one day and they will become a heartache that no woman ever has to suffer again.

In the following chapters we'll discuss the types of molar pregnancies that exist as well as the risk factors for developing them and the chances of having another one in a subsequent pregnancy. The chances of it happening again, incidentally, are actually very low - around 1-2%. We'll also go over any complications that can arise even after the molar pregnancy has been removed and what treatment options are available.

Lastly, we'll talk about recovering from the molar pregnancy, physically and emotionally, and moving forward with subsequent pregnancies. We'll offer plenty of tips to get you started on the road to recovery and to conceive again if and when you are ready. There are lots of ways that you can prepare your body and mind for a new pregnancy and increase both you and your partner's fertility and we'll help you form a plan of action to get you motivated.

Introduction

The chances are that unless you've experienced a molar pregnancy yourself (or know someone who has) it is not a term that you are familiar with. It is a very rare condition and not something that most women experience. Unfortunately, it *is* something that many women still suffer through and it can be an overwhelming loss. In many cases, the woman thought she had a completely "ordinary" pregnancy that was progressing as normal. In other cases, the woman didn't realize she was pregnant at all and is then suddenly met with the news that not only is she pregnant, but that she will probably need to have a procedure to terminate the pregnancy.

Molar pregnancies are a type of gestational trophoblastic disease (GTD), a group of disorders that lead to an abnormal production of placental (trophoblastic) tissue. The hydatidiform mole (the term is used interchangeably with "molar pregnancy") accounts for 80% of the cases of GTD, according to Healthline.com. Molar pregnancies can come with a whirlwind of emotions and feelings, not to mention symptoms and physical strains that can sometimes take weeks (or even months depending on the treatment) to recover from.

In a healthy pregnancy, an embryo is formed within the egg sac. However, in a molar pregnancy there might not be an embryo at all. The pregnancy is simply not a viable one. Sometimes, there is a natural miscarriage of the pregnancy but in many cases it must be terminated for the sake of the woman's health. Although this is difficult enough, occasionally tissue can remain behind and can even turn cancerous. While 90% of molar pregnancies are benign, the other 10% can turn to malignant GTD in different forms which can cause severe health complications for the woman later on.

Luckily, the cure rate for molar pregnancies is very high, almost 100%. In addition, although sometimes further treatment is needed to treat a persistent form of the disease, even when the disease has spread to other parts of the body it is highly treatable.

Although a molar pregnancy can be a heartbreaking experience, and be both physically and emotionally painful, there is still hope for future pregnancies. In fact, less than 2% of the women who were affected by molar pregnancies in the past experience them again, meaning that 98% of women do go on to have normal pregnancies that result in healthy live births.

Chapter 1: What is a molar pregnancy?

In a normal pregnancy, the body releases an egg during ovulation. The egg travels down the fallopian tube and waits around for up to 24-36 hours. If intercourse occurs within that time period, and sperm reaches the egg, it can be fertilized. The genes and gender are determined at time of fertilization. During that time, if a sperm fertilizes it, the egg starts dividing into a lot of different cells as it begins traveling back up into the uterus. Once it reaches the uterus, it attaches itself to the wall.

In a molar pregnancy, something goes awry in this process, right from the beginning. It is important to note that the issue is *not* something that either parent had anything to do with, but is something that occurred immediately upon conception.

A molar pregnancy is a type of gestational trophoblastic disease (GTD). Gestational trophoblastic disease is a tumor that develops from the trophoblast, which is the layer of cells surrounding the core of the fertilized egg. The trophoblast helps the egg attach to the uterine wall and later forms the placenta. The main kinds of gestational trophoblastic diseases are:

- hydatidiform mole (complete or partial);
- invasive mole;

- choriocarcinoma
- placental-site trophoblastic tumor

The most common form of GTD is the hydatidiform mole, also known as a molar pregnancy. It is essentially a noncancerous, or benign, growth that develops within the uterus at the time of conception when there should have been a normal pregnancy.

Molar pregnancies occur when an extra set of paternal chromosomes occur in a fertilized egg. This happens during the fertilization process and changes what would ordinarily go on to be the placenta into a collection of cysts (or abnormal growths) inside the uterus. In a regular pregnancy, the placenta would develop along with the growing fetus and feed the baby. Instead, in a molar pregnancy, there is an over-production of this tissue and it has no real purpose.

A molar pregnancy, sometimes simply referred to as a "mole" in its abbreviated form of hydatidiform mole, does not always involve a developing embryo. In addition, the growth of the tissue matter can be extremely quick in comparison to normal fetal growth. (This is actually one of the first "warning signs" that something is wrong. We'll discuss the other signs in a moment.) If you were to look at the tissue, it would appear to be a large cluster of grape-like material.

Human Chorionic Gonadotrophin (hCG) is the pregnancy hormone that is present in the blood after conception. It is produced by the cells that make up the placenta. When you take a pregnancy test, this is the hormone that the test is searching for that will make it come up either a positive or a negative. However, it generally takes around 3-4 weeks from the first day of your last period for the levels of hCG to be high enough to be detected by the tests. In a molar pregnancy, since the pregnancy can progress so rapidly, the hCG can elevate very quickly - too quickly given the stage of the pregnancy - and the numbers can be a lot higher than what they should be. This is another sign that something might be "wrong" with the pregnancy and is a culprit behind many of the symptoms.

When it comes to molar pregnancies, there are two main kinds. These are referred to as "complete" and "partial."

What is a complete molar pregnancy?

A complete molar pregnancy has the parts of the placenta (or sometimes a whole placenta) present, but you won't find any baby attached to it. It forms when the sperm fertilizes an empty egg. The "pregnancy" is essentially just a mass of tissue. A baby doesn't get the chance to materialize since the egg sac is empty.

The placenta itself will continue to grow in a complete molar pregnancy and the pregnancy hormone, hCG, will be produced. If you were to have an ultrasound, though, only a placenta would show up - not a developing fetus. If left alone, the matter could continue to grow. The tissue should be removed immediately in order to ensure that it's all been taken out to help prevent later health complications.

What is a partial molar pregnancy?

In a partial molar pregnancy, the mass that is formed contains abnormal cells and at least parts of an embryo. However, the embryo is not a healthy or viable one and cannot be "saved." It will have strong defects. The developing tissue will be overwhelmed by the abnormal mass very quickly, given its swift growth period.

Twins and molar pregnancies

In some cases, twins can be affected by a partial molar pregnancy. This is sometimes referred to as "twinning" and is very rare. In the UK, less than 1% of molar pregnancies involve twins, according to Cancer Research UK (www.cancerresearchuk.org). In the United States, molar pregnancies that occur alongside a healthy fetus occur in about 1 in 22,000 – 1 in 100,000 pregnancies. When twins are concerned, one embryo develops normally but the other is a molar pregnancy. In this scenario, there are several different things that can happen and every case is unique.

In some cases, the molar pregnancy may overtake the healthy embryo and the pregnancy would have to be terminated. In other cases, the molar pregnancy may not overtake the healthy embryo but the mole may cause a lot of excess bleeding or another problem, such as preeclampsia, and the pregnancy could then end too early and cause a termination of the viable twin.

However, there have been cases of pregnancies in which the viable twin was delivered successfully and the mole was simply removed upon birth. These pregnancies were treated by specialists and considered extremely high risk. No two cases are ever alike and must be treated individually.

Twinning with a complete mole and a viable fetus with a healthy placenta has also been reported. The viable fetus has gone on to be born as a healthy infant and has survived. However, in most cases women with a simultaneous molar and normal gestation are at higher risk for developing persistent trophoblastic disease and metastasis. As a result, their doctor sometimes recommends that they terminate the pregnancy. Certainly, the woman may choose to continue the pregnancy as long as she is stable and relatively healthy. It is important that she is informed of the risk of her maternal morbidity, though. This is something that must be decided on a personal basis. In this kind of situation, pre-natal genetic diagnosis, usually by chorionic villus sampling or amniocentesis, is usually carried out in order to assess the fetus' karyotype (the number and appearance of chromosomes in the cells' nucleus).

In a study published by The Lancet in 2002, 77 twin pregnancies were studied that were made up of one viable embryo and one complete mole. The study was carried out to determine the risks to both mother and child should the pregnancy continue to full gestation, versus the early termination of the pregnancy.

Out of the 77 women, 24 of them opted to have their pregnancies terminated. Although 53 women did initially continue on, 2 more also had to terminate theirs eventually due to preeclampsia and 23 had miscarriages before 24 weeks gestation. The outlook, however, was overall very positive since out of the pregnancies that extended into the third trimesters, 28 pregnancies lasted for 24 weeks or more and there were 20 live births (Sebire, 2002).

In this study, it was also determined that the women who had both a viable embryo and mole were at a high risk of miscarriage. Still, close to 40% of those who continued with their pregnancies had live births, a hopeful outlook.

What is an ectopic pregnancy?

An ectopic pregnancy is similar to a molar pregnancy only in that it is not a viable pregnancy. It is also more common and happens to as many as 1 in 50 pregnancies in the United States, according to the March of Dimes' website. In the United Kingdom, the NHS estimates as many as 1 in 90 pregnancies is an ectopic one, which is about 10,700 pregnancies per year.

In an ectopic (which means "out of place") pregnancy, the fertilized egg remains in the fallopian tube (more than 95% of the time) or sometimes becomes attached to the outside of the uterine wall (Burd, 2013). It can also be called a tubal pregnancy. It is a very serious condition and can even be life threatening.

Most of the time, ectopic pregnancies occur right away and they are generally discovered within the first few weeks of pregnancy. Sometimes, the pregnancy will terminate itself and be released naturally through a miscarriage. In rare, serious cases the fallopian tube that is affected (if the pregnancy is in the fallopian tube) can rupture and this can require emergency surgery to remove the tube.

Unlike in a molar pregnancy, in an ectopic pregnancy the hCG levels tend to be low instead of very high.

Symptoms of an ectopic pregnancy can include:

- Vaginal bleeding
- Sharp stomach cramping
- Dizziness
- Weakness
- Lower stomach pain
- Pain the neck or shoulder

If your fallopian tube ruptures then the pain could be bad enough that you pass out. The bleeding could also be enough to cause hemorrhaging. It is important to contact your doctor, or go to the E.R. or A&E, if you experience any of these symptoms since your fertility (and even your life) could be at risk.

In most cases of ectopic pregnancies, the cause is unknown. There is only about a 10% chance that it will happen again in subsequent pregnancies though.

The chances of having a successful pregnancy in the future can be dependent upon on the overall health of your fallopian tubes. Sometimes, the tube affected by the ectopic pregnancy must be removed in a surgery called a salpingectomy. This does not tend to hinder fertility, however, as long as the ovary connected to the remaining fallopian tube is producing eggs. The NHS reports that 65% of women realize a successful pregnancy within 18 months of suffering an ectopic pregnancy.

There are certain risk factors that put some women at higher risks for ectopic pregnancies than other women. These include:

- A prior ectopic pregnancy
- Earlier operations on the fallopian tubes
- Drugs used in fertility treatments and those associated with assisted reproductive techniques (such as in vitro fertilization)
- A pregnancy after a failed tubal sterilization
- A history of endometriosis
- Smoking

STDs remain the biggest risk factors for ectopic pregnancies, especially chlamydia. These can cause pelvic inflammatory disease and scarring. When the fallopian tubes scar, the risk of ectopic pregnancy increases.

How common are molar pregnancies?

Molar pregnancies account for around 1 in 1,000-1,500 pregnancies in the United States, making them highly uncommon. The National Health Service (NHS) estimates that 1 in every 600-800 women develop molar pregnancies each year in the United Kingdom.

There are some risk factors, such as maternal age and medical history, which can affect these statistics and these will be discussed in more depth in the next chapter.

It is important to remember that repeated molar pregnancies are very rare. In fact, the chance of having a second molar pregnancy in a subsequent pregnancy is only about 1-2% (1 or 2 in 100), so it is very low, although that percentage does increase to 15-25% for a third pregnancy if you have had two previous molar pregnancies.

The fact that molar pregnancies are not very common is encouraging, especially when it comes to subsequent pregnancies. After all, your chances of it happening again if you want to conceive are low. However, if you are one of the women who develop a mole in the first place, and then go on to develop persistent gestational trophoblastic disease or a malignant form of the disease then the low statistics might not sound as encouraging.

The important thing to remember is that awareness is being raised and studies are being conducted every day in this area. In the future, it is likely that the statistics will only continue to improve.

The positive thing to keep in mind, too, is that even after diagnosis the disease itself is highly treatable with an almost 100% cure rate.

Chapter 2: What causes a molar pregnancy?

Molar pregnancies are caused by abnormally fertilized eggs. A molar pregnancy occurs when there are problems at conception with the chromosomes. This is something that occurs during fertilization, at conception, and is almost certainly a genetic issue. Although there isn't yet a "prevention" or "cure" for it, it isn't due to anything that either partner did wrong.

Under normal circumstances, human cells contain 23 pairs of chromosomes: 23 from the father while the other 23 originate from the mother, totaling 46. However, in complete molar pregnancies, all of the fertilized egg's chromosomes derive from the father. Not long after fertilization occurs, something happens to the chromosomes from the mother's egg and they are either lost or inactivated, perhaps due to an inactive nucleus or no nucleus at all. As a result, the father's chromosomes are copied.

In a complete molar pregnancy, you generally won't see an amniotic sac, fetus, or any kind of regular looking tissue.

When a partial or incomplete molar pregnancy occurs, the mother's chromosomes linger but the father offers two sets of chromosomes. Consequently, rather than having 46 chromosomes, the embryo will have 69. This can occur if the father's chromosomes are copied or if two sperm fertilize the same egg.

If this happens, you might see some regular looking placental tissue surviving around the irregular tissue. The embryo will start developing, so there might even be a fetus or there may just be some fetal tissue or a simple amniotic sac. However, even if there is fetus-type tissue present, generally there are so many defects that it is not viable.

Common risk factors of molar pregnancies

Molar pregnancies are very uncommon. However, there are some risk factors involved that can put some women at a higher risk than others. These include:

Maternal age - According to the University of Michigan Health System's website, a molar pregnancy is more likely to happen to a woman older than age 35 or younger than age 20. Those under the age of 15 are around 20 times more likely than someone aged 20-40 to develop a molar pregnancy, while those over 45 are much more likely than those between the ages of 20-40. The increased risk is mostly for complete molar pregnancies. In cases of partial molar pregnancies, the incidence rates do not change as much (Gestational Trophoblastic Disease (GTD), 2007).

Previous molar pregnancy - If you've had one molar pregnancy, you are more likely to have another. A repeat molar pregnancy happens, on average, in 1 to 2 out of every 100 women in the United States and 1 in 55 for those in the United Kingdom.

Some ethnic groups - Women of Southeast Asian descent appear to have a higher risk of molar pregnancy. Caucasian women are at higher risk in the US than African American women.

A diet low in carotene - One study in 1985 showed that women who had diets low in carotene, a form of vitamin A, had higher rates of complete molar pregnancies. However, no further studies have been conclusive on this.

Use of oral contraceptives - There were studies in the past that indicated that long-term use of oral contraceptives appears to increase the risk of partial molar pregnancies. However, these studies appear to be incomplete. A 1984 study from China did find an increased link between long-term oral contraceptive use and malignant trophoblastic disease prior to conception, but the sample size was very low (only 28 participants).

Smoking - A 1985 Italian study found a correlation between women who smoked and the incidence of molar pregnancies. In this study, 100 women with trophoblastic tumors and 200 controls were studied and it was determined that those who smoked were at a higher risk for developing the disease (La Vecchia C, 1985).

Can a molar pregnancy be prevented?

Molar pregnancies can be disheartening and even frightening. In addition, they can have long-term effects on your health, depending on any complications they might have caused. So is there any way to prevent them?

Unfortunately, at this time, molar pregnancies cannot be "prevented," unless you don't become pregnant at all. It is important to remember that neither you nor your partner did anything wrong to cause the molar pregnancy in the first place. However, early detection is important to finding them sooner rather than later and this can improve your chances of having a healthy subsequent pregnancy and avoiding any health complications.

When it comes to early diagnosis, most physicians familiar with molar pregnancies recommend early ultrasounds performed in subsequent pregnancies. Not only can this help reassure a woman that her pregnancy is progressing normally, but a complete molar pregnancy can often be detected via ultrasound at around 7 or 8 weeks. Unfortunately, partial molar pregnancies are difficult to detect very early since they can appear regular, especially if an embryo (or embryonic tissue) is present.

Some people wonder and question if in vitro fertilization (IVF) and pre-implantation genetic diagnosis can be helpful in preventing molar pregnancies. Although, in theory, pre-implantation should be able to identify molar pregnancies in IVF pregnancies, it is not normally recommended due to its complexity, cost, and risk of complications to the mother. In addition, IVF only results in pregnancy in roughly 25% of cases.

Due to the fact that subsequent molar pregnancies are so low to begin with, IVF screening is only seriously considered an option if the woman experiences multiple molar pregnancies and is experiencing difficulty with conception after trying for a year or longer. Of course, this is something that you would want to discuss with your doctor and fertility specialist. If you have a history of molar pregnancies and miscarriages then IVF might be an option that you want to consider.

In a subsequent pregnancy, some couples request genetic counselling before trying to conceive again. This can be a good way of helping to set their minds at ease, especially if there are any other health concerns they wish to talk about.

Chapter 3: Symptoms of a molar pregnancy

Understanding how to detect the early symptoms of a molar pregnancy is important in finding it and having it diagnosed before it has any negative ramifications on your overall health. Unfortunately, a molar pregnancy can progress along like a normal pregnancy in the beginning and it can be difficult to differentiate it from a healthy one. Still, there are signs that you can look for and being familiar with these is important, especially if you decide to conceive again.

Some of the signs and symptoms of a molar pregnancy can include:

- Dark brown to bright red vaginal bleeding in the first trimester. According to the Women's Cancer Center's page on trophoblastic disease, 80-90% of women with molar pregnancies develop abnormal bleeding (Jeffrey L. Stern, 2007)
- If there isn't bleeding then you might also experience a watery brown discharge
- Severe nausea and vomiting
- The passing of cysts or blood clots that resemble grapes
- Pelvic pain or pressure (rare, but does occur)

Some women experienced symptoms that they can only describe as "vague." Although the feelings are not anything that they can put into words, they just knew that something was wrong and the pregnancy was not progressing in a way that they felt comfortable with. They felt like "something wasn't right" with it.

Likewise, although their morning sickness was bad, in some cases it was so violent that they were unable to function normally and couldn't keep any food down or even go to work. This is consistent with hyperemesis, which is an extreme form of morning sickness and often requires hospitalization.

In addition, other women noticed that their stomachs grew rapidly. This was a sign that was noticeable for some before they even knew they were pregnant - they simply thought they were bloated or retaining water. Or, if they were aware they were pregnant, they may have started wearing maternity clothes very early on and felt a hardening of their stomachs. Later, results would show an enlarged uterus - too big for the stage of pregnancy they were at. Or, the embryo might measure two weeks behind when the woman might know she conceived.

If you experience any signs that may be consistent with a molar pregnancy, contact your doctor. They may notice other signs, which could include:

- Swift uterine growth (the uterus is too big considering the pregnancy's stage). This is present in about 25% of molar pregnancies

- Anemia

- Overactive thyroid (hyperthyroidism). Symptoms of this can include: rapid heartbeat, intolerance to heat, loose stools, warm skin, unexplained weight loss, and mild shaking

- Increased hCG levels

- No fetal movement or heartbeat seen or heard

In addition, because the uterus can expand more quickly than normal, it is not uncommon to feel cramping as well as abdominal swelling.

At first, the symptoms might be typical of what you would experience in any early pregnancy. Eventually, however, you might notice some spotting or even heavier bleeding. The bleeding may be bright red or a brownish discharge. It could be continuous or sporadic, light or heavy. Some women notice this bleeding around 6 weeks into their pregnancies or almost as soon as they become aware that they're pregnant, while others don't see it until they're almost at the end of their first trimester.

It can also be difficult to differentiate this bleeding from a subchorionic hematoma (gathering of blood between the uterine walls and placenta), miscarriage, or even implantation bleeding which is why it is important to report any vaginal bleeding to your doctor. Many women experience light to moderate bleeding throughout their pregnancies and no harmful cause is ever even found and they go on to have perfectly healthy babies.

Preeclampsia

Preeclampsia is a blood pressure-related problem that is specific to pregnancy. It generally occurs after the 20th week in a pregnancy; however, because a molar pregnancy can have symptoms that evolve very quickly, sometimes symptoms similar to preeclampsia can happen as early as the first trimester when a mole is concerned.

Symptoms of preeclampsia include sudden high blood pressure in addition to other issues, such as protein in the urine and swelling of the legs and face. You might also experience headaches that won't go away and feel generally ill.

Although swelling is generally the outward sign of preeclampsia, it's blood pressure that will help determine if you have it - that and a urine test. Your blood pressure measures how hard your blood is pushing against the walls of your arteries. If it is too hard, then you can have high blood pressure (also referred to as hypertension). This is dangerous since it can cause you have to have a heart attack or stroke.

Your blood pressure is shown as two different numbers: the top (systolic) shows the pressure of the heart pumping the blood and the bottom (diastolic) shows the pressure of the heart relaxing and filling up with it. Your blood pressure is high if the top number is greater than 140 or the bottom is greater than 90. An example of a high blood pressure, for instance, might be 160/70 or 130/97. Both numbers can also be high.

If you experience sudden swelling and weight gain very early in your pregnancy then this could be a sign of a molar pregnancy. It is something that needs to be brought to the attention of your doctor. In other types of pregnancies, women are often able to deliver healthy babies by being put on bed rest and carefully monitored. However in a molar pregnancy it can be especially dangerous because the preeclampsia type symptoms can happen so early.

Theca lutein cysts

Theca lutein cysts are frequently seen in complete molar pregnancies, and only in about 5% of partial moles. Fluid-filled cysts on the ovaries often develop in response to the mole that is present. These ovarian cysts are usually larger than 6 cm in diameter and can cause ovarian swelling. While they can't always be felt when examined physically, they can be seen on ultrasound and show up as black spots.

Some women may notice extra pain or pressure in the ovaries with these cysts. Since the ovaries might be enlarged, there is also an increased risk of torsion (rotation of the ovary). The cysts themselves grow in response to the high levels of beta-hCG.

Once the mole has been removed, cysts will usually degenerate but it can sometimes take several months for them to go away completely.

Hyperemesis gravidarum

Some women experience severe nausea and vomiting which is not the same as morning sickness. In fact, as many as 10% of women with molar pregnancies also get diagnosed with hyperemesis gravidarum which is an extreme form of morning sickness and can cause dehydration and hospitalization. The hyperemesis is probably due to the very high levels of hCG, although it is not an affliction that is only seen in molar pregnancies; it can happen in healthy pregnancies as well.

With morning sickness, a woman might feel queasy and vomit a couple of times a day. Eating a light meal or crackers and taking certain anti-nausea medication will usually help with the nausea. However, hyperemesis is characterized by unrelenting nausea and vomiting and is associated with ketosis (the spilling of ketones into the urine) and weight loss (a drop of up to 5% from pre-pregnancy weight). It can cause electrolytes and acid-base imbalances, dizziness, weakness, depression, nutritional deficiencies, and can even be fatal in rare cases if it is left untreated and leads to severe dehydration.

Additional symptoms of hyperemesis can include:

- Sleep difficulty
- Extreme sensitivity to odors (Hyperolfaction)
- Lack of taste (Dysgeusia)
- Anxiety
- Irritability
- Mood changes
- Impaired concentration
- Renal failure
- Atrophy

- Liver disease - maternal liver disease can be found in almost 50% of all women with hyperemesis
- Depression - in a 2013 study posted by Massachusetts General Hospital's Center for Women's Mental Health it was found that 78% of the 200 women admitted to the study with hyperemesis suffered from either mild, moderate, or severe depression that was not present before the pregnancy or medical condition (Hizli, 2012)

According to a study published in the *Journal of Women's Health* in 2009, additional statistics for hyperemesis include: 36% of women suffer from anemia, 33% from muscle pain, 14% from confusion, 12% from oral bleeding, 36% from mood changes, and 25% from insomnia (Fejzo M, 2009).

Like molar pregnancies, hyperemesis is something that not many people understand and can be emotionally and physically straining. To learn more information, and to find an online support group, visit http://www.helpher.org.

Determining a molar pregnancy

It is important that you let your doctor know if you experience any symptoms that might be synonymous with a molar pregnancy. If something doesn't feel right to you, it is always better to err on the side of caution. Sometimes a woman might feel silly for feeling that something is amiss and believe that calling the physician is overreacting. Although it's true that in most cases there is no reason to be alarmed when it comes to a pregnancy, it is always better to be reassured. A good physician, or midwife, will be understanding and work with you and answer any questions you may have.

If your doctor suspects that you might harbor a molar pregnancy, the first thing he will probably do is order a blood test to measure your hCG levels. This is the pregnancy hormone you carry in your blood and the levels will let your doctor know whether or not you are where you should be in your pregnancy. You should not be surprised if your doctor has you wait a couple of days after he or she does your blood work and then checks you again to see if the hCG levels have changed. In a molar pregnancy, the hCG levels are usually abnormally high and can even double or triple within 24-48 hours and be even higher (although in a healthy pregnancy it is normal for them to increase as well).

In a healthy pregnancy the placenta makes many hormones to support the baby and the mother. In a molar pregnancy, however, there is an overgrowth of the placenta and a large amount of hCG is generated.

BhCG moves through the mother's blood while hCG is removed through the urine. Both of these are measured in the lab using blood and urine samples and they are valuable in determining the diagnosis of molar pregnancies, as well as if the mother is later cured. When there is no trace of the molar pregnancy remaining in the body, the level of BhCG in the blood and hCG in the urine will be very low.

While waiting for the blood and urine tests to come back, your doctor might also do an ultrasound to see if they are able to find an embryo or egg sac within the uterus.

Ultrasounds have come a long way, thanks to modern technology. In later pregnancy, the high-frequency sound waves are directed at the stomach and pelvic tissues. However, in early pregnancy it is usually only possible to see inside the uterus using a transvaginal ultrasound since the uterus and fallopian tubes are closer to the vagina than to the stomach's surface. This device resembles a wand and is inserted into the vagina with gel on the end of it to make it more comfortable. Although you might feel pressure, it's not a painful procedure.

When trying to determine a molar pregnancy, ultrasounds can detect several different things, depending on the kind of molar pregnancy you might have. In a complete molar pregnancy (which can be detected as early as 8 weeks) an ultrasound might show:

- Lack of embryo or fetus
- Lack of amniotic fluid
- A large cystic placenta that fills the uterus
- Multiple ovarian cysts

When it comes to a partial molar pregnancy, an ultrasound might show:

- A fetus that is not growing
- Low levels of amniotic fluid
- A solid, cystic placenta

As well as an ultrasound, a pelvic exam will be performed. These can be uncomfortable and you might feel pressure. It may be necessary for your doctor to perform one, however, to check on the size of your uterus. A pelvic exam can reveal a uterus that is bigger or smaller than it is supposed to be or enlarged ovaries.

If a molar pregnancy is detected through blood work, a pelvic exam and an ultrasound, then your doctor will probably check for other related medical issues. These can be, but are not limited to:

- Preeclampsia
- Hyperthyroidism
- Anemia

Depending on your symptoms, your doctor might also order a CT or MRI of your abdomen, blood clotting tests, and kidney and liver function tests. It is important to be thorough and rule out any other problems that might be going on as well.

hCG levels in a molar pregnancy

A lot will be said about hCG levels. If you've been diagnosed with a molar pregnancy or trophoblastic disease then having your hCG tested will become routine. Knowing what the numbers mean is important.

In most molar pregnancies, the levels will be a lot higher than they should be. To give you an example, by the 6th week of pregnancy (gestational age) hCG should be somewhere around 1,080 – 56,500 mIU/ml. However, a woman with a molar pregnancy might have her blood drawn and find that her levels are 90,000 mIU/ml.

As the pregnancy progresses, the hCG levels will get higher (from 7 – 8 weeks they should be from 7, 650 – 229,000 mIU/ml) but then drop again toward the middle of the second trimester.

A low hCG level can mean any number of things and should be rechecked within 48-72 hours to see how the level is changing.

In a molar pregnancy, the woman's numbers might be twice what they should be and then either double or triple every 24 hours. Still, the numbers should increase in a normal pregnancy anyway so it is not just the hCG levels that should be looked at in the first trimester. The doctor should also take symptoms into consideration, as well as the ultrasound. Unfortunately, most ultrasounds won't show much until after about 7-8 weeks and this can be very stressful, especially if you've already had a mole in the past and are in a subsequent pregnancy.

Where hCG levels will be really important will be after the pregnancy has ended. When you are no longer pregnant and the mole has been removed, your number should be negative, or very close to it. Some women, however, continue to see 3,000 mIU/ml or more and sometimes that will double within a week.

Official diagnosis

Although your physician can determine a molar pregnancy through ultrasound in most cases, the official diagnosis is sometimes not given until after the placenta and surrounding tissue have been sent off to a pathologist. This, of course, only happens after the tissue has been extracted and the pregnancy has been terminated.

A pathologist can examine the placenta and any other tissue under a microscope. By then, you should be well on your way to recovery.

In quite a few states in the US and Canada, it is a legal requirement that the tissue be examined by a pathologist. However, it is not a legal requirement in the UK - only a guideline of the Royal College of Obstetricians and Gynaecologists.

Chapter 4: After the diagnosis

Unfortunately, since a molar pregnancy isn't a viable pregnancy, it isn't possible to move forward with it as you would a normal, healthy pregnancy. It can't be saved. In most cases, especially in a complete molar pregnancy, there isn't even an embryo present. The molar pregnancy, and all tissue related to it, must be removed in order to prevent any complications to the mother. This must be done as soon as the molar pregnancy is diagnosed. Around 90% of women who have a molar pregnancy removed require no further treatment.

In some cases, the mother might find that her pregnancy naturally ends in a miscarriage, perhaps before she even realized she was pregnant. Should this occur, the physician would be able to send the tissue off for testing to determine whether or not the pregnancy was, indeed, a mole. Although the idea of collecting the tissue might be a traumatizing one, it is important to try to collect a sample of it if possible, especially if a molar pregnancy was suspected. However, if this isn't a possibility then your physician might still order a dilation and curettage (D&C as discussed below) to ensure that all traces of the tissue have been eradicated from your body.

This is an uncomfortable procedure but it really is for your own health and safety and is occasionally performed after some miscarriages to ensure that all tissue has been removed.

Dilation and curettage (D&C)

If the pregnancy does not end in a miscarriage, a dilation and curettage (D&C) will most likely be performed. A D&C is usually performed as an outpatient procedure in a hospital by your own OBGYN (or gynecologist if you don't have an OBGYN). This procedure normally takes around 30 minutes to perform. You'll be given local or general anesthesia so you won't actually feel it.

During the procedure you'll lie on your back and your legs will be in stirrups, similar to the position you are in during pelvic exams in your gynecologist's office.

A speculum will be inserted into your vagina in order to clearly visualize your cervix. Your cervix will then be dilated by your physician. A hollow plastic tube will be inserted through the cervix and will suction out the uterus' tissue. Lastly, an instrument shaped like a spoon, called a curette, is used to gently scrape the rest of the tissue from the uterus' walls. Medicine (like oxytocin) is used either during or after the procedure. This causes the uterus to contract, similarly to how it would perform during labor. Uterine contractions help the uterus shrink to its pre-pregnancy size. It is important for this to occur since it helps stop uterine bleeding after the molar pregnancy growth is removed from the body.

When you wake up, you'll feel some discomfort and will probably experience some vaginal bleeding for a couple of days, similarly to what you would experience during a light period. You might also notice some cramping. You should get sent home with some pain medication but paracetemol or Tylenol might help as well if you are just experiencing mild pain. For the first 24 hours you might not feel like doing anything but sleeping, although some women feel okay and are able to carry out light activity.

You may well also have a chest X-ray afterward to see whether any abnormal cells from the molar pregnancy have spread to your lungs. It is rare for these cells to spread to other parts of the body, but if they do, the lungs are the most common site.

Hysterectomy

In rare situations, the molar tissue might be extensive. If this is the case, and you don't have any desire to have future children, then your doctor might talk to you about the option of having a hysterectomy.

In a full hysterectomy, both the ovaries and the uterus are removed. Since the ovaries are removed, and the ovaries are responsible for producing the female hormones (estrogen) in the body, it becomes necessary to take these hormones synthetically. Your doctor will talk to you about hormone replacement therapy (HRT).

You might also consider a partial hysterectomy in which only the uterus is removed. This can be a consideration when the molar pregnancy only affected the uterus. Many women consider this option when they don't want to have their ovaries removed.

Additional treatment

Once the mole and surrounding tissue are removed, your physician will look at your hCG levels again. He or she will then want to monitor your levels of hCG once a week to make sure they're declining – an indication that no molar tissue remains.

Some women find that their levels drop very quickly after the D&C. For instance, before surgery, you might have levels of 400,000 and then within 24 hours drop to 180,000. Within a week it could drop to as low as 80,000 and steadily decrease from there on out.

However, other women find that while their levels originally drop after the D&C, after several weeks they level out and then start to rise again.

You will almost certainly need additional treatment if you continue to have hCG in your blood. Once the levels go down to zero for a few weeks in a row, you may still have to have them checked every month or two for the next year. Since pregnancy makes it so challenging to monitor the levels, your doctor might even advise waiting as long as six months before trying to conceive (TTC) again.

Follow-up is important because it ensures that the molar pregnancy (or mole) has been completely removed. If traces of the mole start to grow again they may possess a cancerous-type threat to other parts of your body.

Phantom GTD

It is very important for the doctor to continue monitoring the hCG levels after the treatment of the mole for several months. He must make sure that the mole is gone and that the disease hasn't returned. Although the blood work is generally pretty accurate, sometimes a woman can have an antibody in her blood that can interfere with the test. When this occurs, the hCG levels can appear higher than they actually are. This phenomenon is referred to as *phantom hCG*. It is estimated that around 3-4% of healthy individuals have human-antimouse antibodies that can actually imitate hCG immunoreactivity and cause this kind of reaction.

Sometimes a woman can be diagnosed with a GTD when she hasn't had one. One symptom of having phantom GTD would be having high levels of blood hCG, yet normal urine levels since the irregular antibodies aren't in the urine.

If the doctor sees that the blood levels of the hCG are high but that the urine isn't, he can order different tests that can tell the difference between the accurate hCG levels and the phantom ones.

Chapter 5: Complications: Persistent GTD and GTN

As previously mentioned, the molar pregnancy itself belongs to a group of disorders. Even once a molar pregnancy has been removed, the tissue can still remain and continue to grow. When this occurs it is called gestational trophoblastic disease (GTD), or sometimes "persistent" gestational trophoblastic disease. (In the United Kingdom and elsewhere it is also called persistent gestational trophoblastic tumor - GTT.) The term is simply a broad one that encompasses both benign and malignant growths within the uterus.

Once a mole has been removed through a D&C, the disease is usually considered treated as long as the hCG levels continue to decrease and eventually reach 0. In more than 80% of cases, it *is* cured and no further treatment is necessary. However, in complete molar pregnancies 10-15% of women may develop persistent gestational trophoblastic disease and require treatment with chemotherapy while around 1% of those with partial molar pregnancies end up needing additional treatment.

In complete molar pregnancies, after a D&C the risks are about 5 times higher for persistent GTD and 2-3 times higher after having a hysterectomy. The greatest risk comes within the first 12 months after the mole has been removed, with most of the cases showing up within 6 months.When the disease persists, but remains benign, it is still referred to as "persistent trophoblastic disease." If it turns malignant, however, it is called gestational trophoblastic neoplasia (GTN).

Symptoms of persistent GTD

For the molar pregnancy to be considered "persistent" and require further treatment, it must either show signs of metastasizing, have increasing hCG levels, have hCG levels that persist for 6 months after the mole has been removed, or see the hCG levels plateau and not move in either direction.

One sign of the first symptoms of persistent GTD is an elevated level of hCG even after the mole has been removed. Sometimes, an invasive mole can make its way deep into the middle layer of the uterine wall and this can lead to vaginal bleeding, also a sign of persistent GTD.

Vaginal bleeding is usually the most common physical sign that women experience. If you do experience abnormal bleeding outside of your regular cycle after your molar pregnancy is removed then it is important to talk to your doctor. They will continue to monitor your hCG levels and will take your bleeding into consideration as well. Some women don't experience the excess bleeding, or else it's very light.

Other women notice that they have abdominal swelling. New cysts can form or you might still have them if you developed them from the molar pregnancy. These can make the stomach swell even more and the cysts can be very painful. They may form on both ovaries or only on one. The cysts can usually be seen on an ultrasound and can rupture. If you experience a ruptured cyst, the pain can be extremely severe and might cause you to feel the need to visit your local E.R. or A&E.

Anemia is another symptom of persistent trophoblastic disease. When you are anemic, your body has a low number of red blood cells. If you are bleeding heavily, or regularly, then your red blood cell count can drop. Since your red blood cells carry oxygen around your body, anemia can make you feel exhausted and even breathless performing simple activities that didn't tire you out in the past.

Even though persistent GTD isn't cancer, it is still treated the same as GTN - with chemotherapy.

Types of GTN

Around 80% of GTD cases are non-cancerous. However, in rare cases, trophoblastic disease can turn into cancer. The good news is that most women who get this kind of cancer are cured with treatment. In the majority of cases, the persistent moles can be treated with chemotherapy, even though they are not actually cancer. However, in rare cases the irregular tissue can spread to other parts of the body and advance to a form of malignant cancer called gestational trophoblastic neoplasia (GTN).

Still, with timely and proper treatment, almost 100% of cases of gestational trophoblastic neoplasia are curable when it hasn't spread outside the uterus. Even when it does spread to other organs, most cases can be cured. It is important to continue to have your hCG levels checked for at least a year, though.

There are four main types of malignant GTNs. These are:

1. Choriocarcinoma

Choriocarcinoma is a malignant form of GTD that can quickly spread throughout the body and requires rapid treatment. It might have started out as a molar pregnancy or it might have formed from tissue that remained in the uterus following a miscarriage. Choriocarcinoma is rare, resulting from only about 1 out of every 25,000 pregnancies in the United States. In the UK, it affects less than 250 women each year - only about 1 in 55,000 pregnancies.

2. Placental-Site Trophoblastic Tumor

Placental-site trophoblastic tumor is a very rare form of the disease. In the United States, they account for around 1% of the disease. In the UK, they only represent around 0.2% of GTNs. It occurs in the uterus at the location where the placenta was attached to the uterus. The tumors infiltrate the muscle layer of the uterus and typically don't spread to other parts of the body. Unlike choriocarcinoma, they aren't very sensitive to chemotherapy. Because the tumor is localized to the uterus, hysterectomies are usually advised in these cases. However, when the disease spreads outside the uterus, high dose chemotherapy is generally used with some success.

3. Invasive mole

An invasive mole is a type of hydatidiform mole that has penetrated the muscle layer of the uterus. These cases are rare and only occur in around 1 pregnancy in 15,000, according to Cancer.org.

4. Epithelioid trophoblastic tumor

Epithelioid trophoblastic tumors (ETT) are very rare types of GTD that can be difficult to diagnose. Only a handful of cases have ever been reported. These used to be referred to as *atypical choriocarcinoma* since the cells resembled choriocarcinoma cells under the microscope. Now, however, it is considered a separate disease.

Choriocarcinoma

Around 2-3% (1 out of 40) of moles can develop into choriocarcinoma. Although only 50% of cases come from hydatidiform moles, 25% follow abortions or tubal pregnancies while 25% occur with full-term gestations.

If the GTD develops into choriocarcinoma then the symptoms can change somewhat and there will be other signs that something is wrong within your body.

Although the problems begin within your uterus, they can spread to other areas. Your lungs are usually the most commonly affected area, which is why your doctor might perform a chest x-ray, but other organs can be affected too.

Symptoms usually depend on where the cancer has spread to and are specific to that area.

Lungs:

- Coughing
- Coughing up blood
- Chest pain
- Trouble breathing

Vagina:

- Nodules
- Heavy, irregular bleeding
- Pain
- Pressure

Stomach:

- Swelling
- Stomach pain

Brain:

- Seizures
- Dizziness
- Headaches
- "Brain fog"
- Vision trouble
- Weakness

Although these symptoms do sound discouraging and even frightening it is important to keep in mind that it's rare that choriocarcinoma ever spreads and that, when it does, it is almost always curable. Even when it does spread to other areas of the body, choriocarcinoma has an extremely high cure rate. At the Charing Cross Trophoblastic Center, it is estimated that survival rate is 80% for cases that have metastasized to the brain (Kenny, 2010).

Placental-Site Trophoblastic Tumor

A placental site trophoblastic tumor (PSTT) can develop from the tissue that forms in the uterus during the molar pregnancy. These develop from the cells, called the trophoblast cells, that are meant to form the placenta. The tumors themselves form once the pregnancy has ended. They don't have to form after a molar pregnancy, although they can. They can also form after a full term pregnancy or miscarriage, or even an abortion. They can crop up months and even years after the pregnancy has ended.

The tumors form in the location where the placenta attached itself to the uterus' lining. The tumors grow slowly and can grow into the muscle. They are very rare. They can grow beyond the uterus and reach other areas of the body, usually preferring the lungs.

Symptoms:

Abnormal vaginal bleeding is the main symptom. Some women also notice that they lose their periods altogether and then experience the abnormal vaginal bleeding. Additional symptoms can include the leakage of milk from the nipple and the development of certain male traits such as excess hair growth on certain body parts and a deeper voice.

Diagnosing:

The doctor will usually send the woman for tests when she reports that her menstrual cycle has stopped or that she is experiencing abnormal bleeding. The tests themselves can include:

- Ultrasounds - an ultrasound might show any irregular area inside the uterus. A Doppler will show that there are more blood vessels then there are supposed to be and this can indicate a tumor.

- Blood work - women with these tumors usually have high levels of hCG. This is caused by the tumor's cells.

- Surgery - the doctor can use a curette to scrape out part of the uterus' lining and send that to the lab. The pathologist can then examine it under a microscope to see if there are any tumor cells in the tissue.

Treatment:

If the tumor is limited to the uterus then surgery is the main treatment. The majority of women opt to have a hysterectomy. As long as it hasn't spread, this should cure it. It is possible to only remove the tumor, especially if you wish to have more children, but the tumor can return. In this situation, it is necessary to continue to have regular blood work done to test the hormone and hCG levels. If any symptoms return or there is any sign of the tumor then a hysterectomy will probably need to be done.

If the tumor has spread to another part of the body then chemo will probably be given after surgery. Chemo is offered until the hCG levels have returned to 0 and then continued for an additional 8 weeks or so to be on the safe side. There will then be follow up treatment that may consist of CT scans, ultrasounds, more blood work, and MRIs. The survival rate is almost 100% if the tumor hasn't metastasized. In a 2009 study conducted in the United Kingdom concerning all women who had been diagnosed with PSTTs, it was discovered that nearly all were cured as long as they were diagnosed within 48 months of their pregnancies (Schmid, 2009).

Invasive mole

An invasive mole can develop from complete or partial moles, but complete moles become invasive more frequently than partial moles. Approximately 1 in 6 cases of a hydatidiform mole can turn into an invasive mole or choriocarcinoma. (Fewer cases turn into the other forms of malignancy.) The chance of developing an invasive mole can increase if:

- There is more than 4 months between the last menstrual period and treatment
- The uterus becomes enlarged
- The woman is more than 40 years old
- There is a prior history of GTD

Since the moles have penetrated the uterus' muscle, a D&C can't completely remove them. Although it is possible for them to go away by themselves, usually more treatment is needed. Some women opt to have a hysterectomy.

Sometimes, a mole that penetrates completely through the uterus' wall can cause excessive bleeding which can be serious.

Even after the removal of a hydatidiform mole, the tumor can metastasize to other parts of the body.

Epithelioid trophoblastic tumors

Epithelioid trophoblastic tumors (ETT)s are very rare. The most common symptom is vaginal bleeding, although other symptoms can occur if it has spread. For instance, if it has spread to the lungs, then there may be shortness of breath or coughing. Vomiting may occur if it spreads to the intestines. The hCG levels are not always elevated or, if they are, they are only slightly so.

ETTs can form in women who have had molar pregnancies, full-term deliveries, and miscarriages. There have been as many as 1 to almost 18 years between the gestation and the diagnosis of the tumor.

Most of the time, the tumors have been found in the lower part of the uterus and most were very small. Unfortunately, ETTs have not responded well to chemotherapy in the past. Instead, surgery has been the best option in treating these types of tumors.

Risk Factors for GTN

The reports of GTD seem to depend on where in the world you live. Still, rest assured, it is rare. In the United States it is around 110-120 per 100,000 pregnancies. For choriocarcinoma, which is the most aggressive form of GTD, it is around 2-7 per 100,000 pregnancies. In the UK, about 0.5% of those with partial molar pregnancies progress to malignant disease, though up to 20% of those with complete molar pregnancies develop them and end up needing treatment such as chemotherapy.

Currently, researchers haven't yet determined why some women develop persistent GTD and why others do not.

About 10-15 out of every 100 women who have had a complete molar pregnancy will develop either persistent trophoblastic disease or a choriocarcinoma, and will need treatment with chemotherapy. For those who have had a partial mole, the risk is only 1%.

Additional risk factors include:

- A pre-evacuation uterine size that was greater than gestational age or bigger than 20 weeks gestation

- The presence of theca-lutein cysts that are bigger than 6 cm

Tests for discovering persistent GTD & metastasis

Since diagnosing GTN can be complicated, more testing is sometimes necessary to ensure that everything has been covered. In addition, it is also important to determine whether or not the disease has metastasized. Some of the tests that can be used to further find and diagnose GTN can include the following:

Pelvic exam: A physical exam may be performed of the uterus, vagina, rectum, and ovaries. This is carried out to feel the shape, size, and position of the uterus and to check the vagina and cervix for indications of disease. A Pap test is normally conducted as well to check for cancerous cells. An exam of the rectum might be carried out to check for any irregular areas in that location.

Lumbar puncture: A lumbar puncture, also called a spinal tap, is used to collect cerebrospinal fluid (CSF) from the spinal column and can check for signs of cancer. This procedure is done by inserting a needle into the spinal column.

Blood chemistry studies: Blood chemistry studies take a blood sample to measure the amounts of certain substances that are released into the blood by organs and tissues. If there is an abnormal amount of a substance it can be a sign of disease in the organ or tissue that makes it.

Serum tumor marker test: In this test a sample of blood is checked to measure the amounts of certain substances that are made by tumor cells, organs, or tissues. This can be connected to particular types of cancer when it is discovered in increased levels. Often referred to as "tumor markers", in GTD the blood is checked for beta human chorionic gonadotropin levels.

Urinalysis: Your urine might be tested to see if you are passing any protein or bacteria or to check your b-hCG levels.

Chest x-ray: A chest x-ray can show the doctor whether or not there are any signs of cancer within your lungs and if the disease has spread to this area. Usually, if the GTD is going to spread, the lungs are the first organs to be affected.

Liver scan: A scan of the liver, using an ultrasound in most cases, can show if the disease has spread there. In addition, bloodwork can show whether or not the liver is functioning properly and this can be a sign that further examination of the liver is needed.

CT scan: The persistent disease will usually call for a CT scan of the pelvis, stomach, and even the brain. This may be in addition to the ultrasound. The results of the CT scan show if the disease is going to be classified as nonmetastatic or metastatic.

CT scans and MRIs can be helpful if there is a mole that has metastasized to the lungs or in cases of persistent gestational trophoblastic disease or choriocarcinoma.

Chapter 6: Treatment of Persistent GTD and GTN

Chemotherapy is the treatment of choice for both persistent GTD and if the tumor has become malignant. In some cases, if the tumor doesn't respond well to chemo or if the woman doesn't want to have any more children and the tumor is contained within the uterus, then a hysterectomy will probably be offered and that might be enough to cure the disease. However, in most cases chemo will be the first line of defense and it usually works.

Talking to your doctor

You'll want to make sure you are on the same page as your doctor, but you'll also want to ensure that you understand everything that's going on as well. The following is a list of questions that you might want to ask about your condition so that you understand some of the decisions that are going to be made.

What kind of GTD do I have?

Is my cancer contained within my uterus? Has it spread elsewhere? Where else is it located?

Can my cancer's stage be determined? What does staging mean?

What is my prognostic score?

Do you have any personal experience treating this disease?

Are there any centers nearby that specialize in the treatment of this?

Can you tell me my treatment choices?

Are there any clinical trials available?

Is there one kind of treatment choice that might reduce the risk of reappearance more than another kind?

What are the side effects and risks of the different treatments?

How will I be monitored?

What do you think my prognosis is?

Is there anything I can do to get myself ready for my treatment?

What will my recovery be like?

When will I be ready to return to work?

When will I be ready to resume sexual intercourse?

What are the chances that the cancer will return?

Will I have a specialist in gynecologic oncology?

If I seek treatment will I still be able to have a normal pregnancy later?

When will I be able to try to conceive again?

Staging

It is important to determine whether the disease, or tumor, has remained in the uterus or if it has spread to other parts of the body. In some places, this is referred to as the "staging." This step is essential since the tests and scans let the doctors know what kind of treatment will suit you best.

The staging system is called the FIGO (International Federation of Gynecology and Obstetrics) staging system. It scores the risk factors to determine which treatment will work best for you by using a numbering system for the stage and risk factor score.

Some of the questions included in the FIGO staging system include the mother's age, the number of months since the pregnancy, the size of the largest tumor, the number of metastases found and if chemotherapy has failed in the past or been used with success.

After your molar pregnancy is removed, if your hCG levels go back to normal and stay there, you won't be assigned a stage. You'll still receive follow-up care for up to a year but you probably won't need any further treatment as long as your hCG levels continue to show a zero.

There are essentially 4 main stages, with Stage 1 being an early tumor and Stage 4 being advanced.

Stage 1:

This is the earliest stage of GTD when the tumor is still limited to the uterus and doesn't spread outside of it.

Stage 2:

The tumor has spread outside the uterus and is now in the surrounding areas.

Stage 3:

The GTD has spread to the lungs and may also be in the areas around the uterus.

Stage 4:

The disease has spread to other parts of the body and is considered very serious and advanced.

Risk factors

Part of your treatment options will depend on your risk factors. When you are diagnosed with GTD your medical team will take a look at certain risk factors and these will help them decide which chemotherapy treatment and drugs are optimal. These risk factors include:

Age: The younger you are, the lower your score is.

The kind of pregnancy you had: A molar pregnancy is considered low risk while an abortion or miscarriage is considered a slightly higher risk and a full term pregnancy is given a higher score.

The time between the end of a pregnancy and your diagnosis: If there was less than 4 months there is a low score and if there was more than a year then a higher score is given.

hCG level in the blood: The higher the level of hCG in the blood, the greater the score.

The amount the tumor has spread: The more the tumor has spread in your body, the higher score you are given.

Affected body parts: Body parts given a low score include the lungs and vagina. Spleen and kidneys get a slightly higher score while the brain and liver get the highest.

Tumor size: The bigger the tumor is, the higher the score it receives.

Prior chemotherapy: Any history with chemotherapy for your GTD raises your score.

Once your score has been tallied, you are then placed into one of two groups. One is considered low risk and one high risk. The low risk group scored 6 or less while the high risk group scored 7 or more. If you scored 7 or more then it means that the doctor believes you are in need of additional treatment.

Chemotherapy treatment

Chemotherapy is the main treatment option for malignant GTD, as well as for benign. Chemo is considered very effective for this. It may be taken by pill form, or by a needle in the vein or muscle. Some women are able to have a few chemotherapy treatments and are considered cured very quickly. These treatments are done by injections into the muscle, usually the buttocks. If you are in need of additional chemotherapy treatment, you may get them by intravenous treatment. Around 80% of those who need chemotherapy treatment after a molar pregnancy are in the low risk group and are able to receive chemo by injection.

For those in the high risk group who must receive chemo intravenously, then treatment becomes more serious. Sometimes, the GTD can even spread to the brain. This is very rare but if it happens then you might need chemo injected into the fluid around your spinal cord. This is referred to as intrathecal chemotherapy.

Generally speaking, the chemotherapy is usually well tolerated without any long-term side effects. Exhaustion and nausea are the most reported issues.

You may be able to receive treatment at your local hospital or you might need to visit a specialist center, depending on where you live. At the beginning of your treatment, you might have to stay at your hospital for as long as a week to see how you adjust to the chemo.

The amount of time you have to stay there depends on the treatment. You'll usually stay for at least a week and then return every week or so for around 3-6 months for additional treatments. The rest of the treatments will be done as an outpatient. It is not uncommon to feel sick with the chemo treatments, although every person reacts to them in a different way.

After chemo treatment, follow-up by measuring the level of hCG in blood will continue until the hormone level is normal for 3 weeks. It will then continue every month for 12 months, or 24 months for those with Stage 4 disease. It is important that you avoid getting pregnant during that time. If you conceive within that time you have an increased risk of miscarriage, especially if you received multiple chemotherapeutic agents. In addition, if you get pregnant before follow-up is finished, it might be hard to see a tumor setback.

Around 10-15% of women with high-risk malignant GTD can develop drug resistance after extended exposure to chemotherapy. These women generally consist of those who have Stage 4 disease that involves organs like the brain and bowels. However, these days there are specifically designed chemotherapy treatments that have been shown to be successful against other cancers and are being used successfully in many of these cases as well.

Methotrexate for Trophoblastic Cancer

Methotrexate is one medication (a form of chemotherapy) that is sometimes used to stop the growth of rapidly reproducing cells, like fetal cells or cancer cells. It is commonly the drug of choice for treating trophoblastic disease that only affects the uterus.

The success rate for Methotrexate is considered high, with about 90% of trophoblastic cancer being cured - as long as it is confined within the uterus and hasn't spread outside of it.

The medication is taken as injections into the buttocks. It is followed with Folinic Acid (not the same as folic acid), which is taken orally within 24 hours after each injection. This protects the internal organs from damage that can arise from the Methotrexate.

After each course of Methotrexate women will generally have blood work drawn. This will check for your liver functions, blood count, blood platelets, hemoglobin, and hCG hormones. Your test results will determine whether or not you can continue the Methotrexate for another cycle.

While on the medication, it is important to drink plenty of water. This will help flush out the toxins. Water is the best hydration but if you find that you can't tolerate water well then juice will also work okay, followed by tea. If you find that you are having trouble keeping anything down then you might get to the point where you need to drink whatever you can stomach, just as long as you can drink something.

Hair loss is one of the most devastating side effects that women worry about when it comes to chemotherapy treatments and it is something that can occur, although it doesn't tend to happen with Methotrexate.

Surgery and radiation

Sometimes women end up needing to have surgery, most commonly a hysterectomy. This may happen if:

- Their GTD doesn't react to the chemo
- The GTD is causing massive vaginal bleeding

It isn't often that doctors resort to radiation for GTD. Chemo is usually the treatment of choice since it is so effective. However, if it spreads to other parts of the body then your doctor might opt to use radiation treatment for that area, especially if it occurs in the brain and lungs and if it doesn't respond well to chemo.

Hysterectomy

In a hysterectomy, the uterus is removed. As previously mentioned, it is an option for those with hydatidiform moles who do not want to have any more children, but it is not a decision to be made lightly since it is not one that can be reversed. Luckily, less than 5% of women need a hysterectomy for treatment, even when the disease has turned malignant.

A hysterectomy is one of the standard treatments for women with placental-site trophoblastic tumors and epithelioid trophoblastic tumors. When the uterus is removed, it ensures that all of the tumor cells in the uterus are also removed. This includes any cells that might have penetrated the muscle layer (myometrium) and buried into it. Unfortunately, due to the fact that some tumor cells could have spread outside the uterus, having a hysterectomy does not ensure that all tumors cells are eradicated. It can, however, reduce the ensuing risk of persistent trophoblastic disease by as much as 50%.

During most hysterectomies, unless otherwise specified, the ovaries are left behind. Unless there are cysts on the ovaries, the ovaries will remain and continue producing estrogen. The ovaries might still remain even if there are cysts on them, but your doctor should talk about your options in this situation.

There are 3 different types of surgeries that can be used:

Abdominal hysterectomy: the uterus is removed through an incision in the front of the abdomen. The incision is either made across the bikini line, horizontally, or vertically across the abdomen. This generally requires a longer recovery time and is done when the uterus might be enlarged and can't be removed any other way.

Vaginal hysterectomy: if the uterus isn't too big, it can be separated and removed through the vagina. A small cut can be made in the abdomen and a laparoscope inserted to help with the surgery. This is called a laparoscopic-assisted vaginal hysterectomy. Since a large abdominal incision isn't involved, recovery is usually faster than with an abdominal hysterectomy. This type of surgery is generally not used if your doctor suspects any kind of cancer present within the ovaries, uterus, or cervix.

Laparoscopic assisted vaginal hysterectomy (LAVH): several small holes are made in the stomach and long, thin instruments are inserted into them to perform the surgery. The uterus is removed through a small hole made in the vagina. Recovery is usually fast.

For all of these surgeries, you can count on being either asleep (under general anesthesia) or sedated and numbed below the waist (under regional anesthesia). Most women remain in the hospital for up to 5 days with an abdominal hysterectomy. You can count on total recovery time taking around 4-6 weeks. With a vaginal hysterectomy hospital stay is about 1-2 days with a recovery time of 2-3 weeks. Recovery time is similar for a laparoscopic hysterectomy.

The major drawback for a hysterectomy is that you will no longer be able to have children. It is common to experience pain after a hysterectomy. Some women have a lot of pain, but it can be managed with medication. Complications are rare but can include:

- Reactions to anesthesia
- Excessive bleeding
- Infection
- Damage to the urinary tract or intestine

- Nerve damage
- Vomiting

In addition to a physical recovery from a hysterectomy, there is an emotional recovery that many women don't consider until after they've had the procedure. A hysterectomy means that you will be unable to have any more biological children in the future. Some women also see this as saying goodbye to a part of what makes them female, even though they still possess all of their outwardly physical traits and continue to produce female hormones.

It is not uncommon to feel sad, depressed, and even angry after having a hysterectomy. The website Hyster Sisters (www.hystersisters.com) is a good place to find support and additional information about hysterectomies and offers a good online forum from other women who have been through the procedure.

Although surgery does eliminate the disease inside the uterus, it doesn't remove the disease that could have spread anywhere else. To be on the safe side, blood hCG levels will continue to be regularly monitored. If they remain the same or start to increase, chemotherapy may be suggested.

Chapter 7: Recovering from the emotional strain

Coping with the loss of your pregnancy can be very difficult. Not only do you have to deal with the emotions that come with the loss of your pregnancy, but it can be very challenging to cope with the physical aspects of your loss as well.

In addition, finding out that you have a molar pregnancy at all can be frightening. Being surprised by the news of what you thought was a normal pregnancy and then discovering that you now have to face a serious health scare can be overwhelming. As with anyone who has suffered a pregnancy loss, you are dealing with the loss of your pregnancy, but in this situation, you are also looking at an atypical condition that most people haven't heard of and you are most likely concerned for your health.

You will probably experience a lot of different feelings with your loss. It is common to feel fear, sadness, guilt, anxiety, and numbness. At the same time, you will almost certainly also have moments when you are not feeling any of those things and you feel happy, elated, and even laugh. Those moments might shock you and even make you feel guilty later when you look back on them. Of course you have nothing to feel guilty about.

Grieving

You will almost certainly feel sad about your loss though that is probably just the tip of the iceberg as far as where your feelings start. Even though, by most standards, it can be considered an "early loss", it is natural to grieve the end of your pregnancy.

Even when there isn't an embryo present, and there wasn't an opportunity for it to develop into a child, you are still grieving the end of a specific hope and dream. Many women discover that they are grieving the dreams, plans, and hopes that they had of being pregnant and these losses can be very significant ones and huge disappointments.

If you weren't aware that you were pregnant then you might be met with the news that you were and that it was a molar pregnancy all at the same time. This can be a shock to your system, both emotionally and physically, and hard for you to take in. If you *were* aware that you were pregnant and you had already started making plans for your future then you now have to take the time to adjust to your new reality – one without the baby.

Grief is strange and everyone grieves differently. It is important to remember that grief isn't linear. Although there are "stages" of grief (anger, depression, denial, etc.) you don't move through them, one by one, until you've completed them. Instead, you can stay in one for a while, move on to another, and jump back into a previous one again. Be gentle with yourself and give yourself plenty of time to be sad and angry and experience the emotions you need to feel in order to process what you are going through.

It can also be helpful to talk to other people. Support groups and counsellors can be invaluable. Many hospitals have pregnancy loss groups and in these you might find others you can reach out to. If you don't feel comfortable doing this in person then you might feel better in an online forum where you are more anonymous.

According to the standard Kubler-Ross grieving model, the stages of grief are as follows:

Denial. In the beginning, it might be difficult to understand what has happened, especially if you didn't know you were pregnant. You might be in shock.

Bargaining. Once you get the news that you may have a molar pregnancy, you might enter the bargaining stage. At this point, you might yourself bargaining with your body, or even your doctor, and promising that you'll take care of yourself and your baby as long as things "get better."

Guilt. You may wonder if the molar pregnancy was your fault or if you could have done something to have prevented it from happening.

Anger. You might find yourself angry at your doctor, your partner, or yourself. You might even be angry at the unfairness of the whole situation and even at the mole.

Depression. At this stage, you might find yourself exhibiting sighs of depression. These can include changes in the way you eat and sleep, loss of interest in normal activities, and difficulty concentrating and making regular decisions.

Acceptance. Eventually, you'll move on into acceptance. This doesn't mean that you are okay with your loss at all. It just means that you have found a new way of living with your "new normal" and that you are functioning with your loss.

You might also experience:

Envy. You might find yourself jealous when you see other pregnant women. Everywhere you look, you see babies and other expecting families and wonder why those can't be you.

Yearning. You could have feelings of longing and desire to be with the baby you never had. You may even find yourself thinking about the baby and wondering what he or she would look like and imagining the baby aging.

It can take as long as two years to go through the roughest parts of the grieving process. Even after the time has gone by, you can still expect to experience those pangs of grief every now and then. You'll probably have triggers, perhaps on certain anniversaries or maybe when you see a newborn baby or another pregnant woman.

Communicating with others in your life

One of the hardest things you might find yourself dealing with is other people. Although well-meaning friends, family members, and co-workers want to be helpful, some of them can really cross the line and say things that can be incredibly hurtful.

Unless they've been through it themselves, not everyone can understand a pregnancy loss. Some people just can't wrap their minds around the fact that a woman can be so attached to a child that she never met and there are many people who really don't consider an embryo a baby, especially in the case of a complete molar pregnancy where the embryo wasn't present.

You might hear such comments as:

> "At least it was an early miscarriage so you didn't have time to get attached to it."

> "At least it wasn't a real baby."

> "Babies are really expensive anyway."

> "You can always have another one."

Some of these are going to sound very mean-spirited while others are simply ignorant.

Many of your friends are going to try to help and ask you what you need and what they can do for you. The problem with that is going to be that you might not know what you need and vocalizing those needs may not be easy. Simply telling them to visit and hang out with you can be enough. Ask them to come around, watch a movie, eat dinner with you. That can be enough.

Don't be surprised if some people don't want to talk about your loss. They might think that bringing it up will make you sad and upset. Ignoring your loss may not be rudeness on their part, but respect. On the other hand, if talking about your loss makes you feel upset, then feel free to change the subject if someone brings it up. You ultimately need to do what's best for you.

If friends want to help:

If friends do come around and offer to help, and they don't know what to do, here are some things that might be helpful…

Send someone to the store for groceries.

Send someone to the store for "thank you cards." Have them fill them out so that all you have to do is sign them.

Ask a few friends to make some dinners, casserole style, that can be frozen. That way, all you have to do is put them in the microwave.

Invite a few people over for movie night. No conversations needed; just some movies and friends.

Ask someone to box up any reminders of the pregnancy; perhaps an early baby gift or the ultrasound picture. You might not want to get rid of these, but having them around at the moment might be too sad.

If needed ask someone to update your social media sites for you, telling everyone that you are okay but not up to chatting yet.

Have someone come around to feed your pets, empty the litter box, take the dog for a walk, etc.

The bottom line is, people feel better when they are useful. Most friends want something to do; they just don't know how to offer. If you give them a chore, they are more than happy to do it. Some friends just feel awkward volunteering.

Talking to your partner

Your partner is probably going to be one of your biggest sources of support. Unfortunately, it can be challenging to meet each other on the same page because men and women often grieve differently.

Since the woman is the one who felt the physical changes during pregnancy it can be difficult for the man to appreciate that aspect of the loss. Some men have trouble connecting to a pregnancy and the idea of a baby until they actually meet their child; which, of course, doesn't mean they're not excited about being pregnant, but does mean that the emotional bond isn't the same.

Often men can feel that they must be "strong" in these types of situations for the sake of their partner - either for reasons that our culture has placed on them or because they simply don't know how to express their emotions. Your partner might not want to burden you with their own emotions, thinking that it might place extra guilt and sadness on you - not realizing that by keeping quiet it's actually creating tension.

It is important to try to communicate with one another in the best way you know how. Talking to your partner, letting each other know how you feel and that you need to talk to one another, and simply being in the same room with one another can help.

If you find that words fail you at times then you might discover that falling back on other forms of communication can be more comfortable. For instance, writing short notes to one another and leaving them on the breakfast table, just letting the other know that you are thinking of them can be a quick way of reminding your partner that you are still there and supporting them.

Finding something to do together, as a couple, might be helpful. One thing that many couples find beneficial is doing something tangible in the name of their loss.

A physical activity or exercise can help people deal with feelings of depression and anxiety. In addition, research has shown that this can offer the chance to work through emotions. Some ideas include:

- Running a marathon
- Planting a tree that will bloom on what would have been your due date
- Picking a name off the Angel Tree at Christmas and buying Christmas presents for a less fortunate child in honor of your pregnancy loss
- Cultivating a memorial garden in honor of your pregnancy

Some women find that the physical aspects of their relationship with their partner are challenged after suffering a loss. Although many women find comfort in a physical relationship, others do not. A lot of men find emotional comfort in sexual release while women find more comfort in cuddling. This can also create tension and a breakdown of communication, especially if both partners are not on the same page.

It can be especially difficult to maintain an active sex life if you've had to undergo surgery, such as a hysterectomy, or are getting chemotherapy treatments that make you feel exhausted and sick. Intercourse may hold no interest.

It is important to remember that caregivers, such as your partner, also suffer the emotional consequences when their loved ones are ill and they often don't have a strong support system to turn to. As a result, they can end up feeling tired, lonely, and guilty for wishing things were "back to normal."

If, after awhile, you are still having communication problems then finding a neutral third party such as a qualified therapist might be advisable. This person can offer advice and might even be able to sit down with both of you and facilitate a discussion in an easy manner. It is usually not recommended that you get a friend involved because that can make the situation awkward for everyone involved, as that person might feel as though they need to "choose sides."

Finding support

Gestational trophoblastic disease, although highly curable, is an emotionally traumatic event, not only because of the pregnancy loss, but also because of the fear of cancer. Treatment of a malignant GTD can drastically affect a woman's self-image as well as her relationships with her partner, friends, and family members. It is not uncommon for women to want to remain "strong" for others but for the sake of their own mental health, it's essential to make use of all available psychological and spiritual support to help you through this challenging period in your life.

It is natural to feel sad and there is no real timeline as to when you should start "feeling better." However, there are certain instances when it is best to call in someone for added support for your own safety. It doesn't mean that you can't handle your grief - it just means that you need a little extra help getting through a rough patch.

If you develop a complication of grief such as disturbing thoughts or depression, contact your doctor or someone you trust. Situations that warrant this include:

- You think about harming yourself
- Your partner threatens to harm you or them
- You begin hearing voices that tell you do things
- You experience a sense of hopelessness that doesn't go away
- You engage in addictive behavior such as consuming too much alcohol or recreational drugs

- You feel like you've been grieving longer than you think you should have been and you want to make a change
- You find it hard to engage in normal activities, such as getting dressed or leaving the house

There are lots of different people who might be able to lend support to you. Your primary care doctor is probably the best person to start with and he or she should be able to give you a referral. Although many women feel comfortable going to a counsellor or psychologist, a psychiatrist might be an option if you feel as though you need someone who can prescribe something for anxiety of depression.

Some community centers, churches or other religious centers, offer support and counselling groups. Some of these are income based, or free if they are support groups, and this can be a good option if you don't have medical insurance.

Other options of mental health professionals as far as who might be able to offer you grief support include:

- Clinical social worker
- Licensed professional counsellor
- General practitioners or family medicine doctors
- Internists
- Physician assistants
- Nurse practitioners

Online forums can be one of the best sources of support, not just for the molar pregnancy but also for any further treatment you might have, such as a hysterectomy, and for any other symptoms you might be experiencing, such as depression, grief, or anxiety. In an online forum you have the opportunity to meet others from all over the world who are going through the same experiences you are, or have already been through them, and understand the challenges you are facing. Details of some of these can be found later in this book.

Some women appreciate the anonymity of online forums while others join them because there are limited support options available in their communities. If you live in a rural area, for instance, it can be difficult to find a grief center or counselling center nearby. If you are recovering from surgery or simply have difficulty leaving the house then it might be hard to travel an hour or more to attend support group meetings. With online support groups, however, you simply need to sign into the group and you have a variety of women right there on the computer, waiting to talk to you - regardless of the hour.

Chapter 8: Recovering from the physical strain

For a while at least, the idea of "recovering" from your molar pregnancy might feel like a strange concept. How can you move on from something that feels like it took the wind out of you? Not only do you have the physical aspects to deal with, but you have the emotional strain of the loss to handle as well. You might find yourself feeling overwhelmed, sad, angry, lost, anxious, hurt, and even numb.

Many women find that they don't have time to feel the emotions they want to because they have to jump right into the treatment without getting the time they need to process the emotions they have. Some women find that they go the first few months in shock and don't feel their real grief until months down the line. Unfortunately, that's about the same time that everyone else in their life has moved on and doesn't want to hear about their loss anymore.

Dealing with the physical strain of a molar pregnancy can be exhausting. Although you might not have carried full term, that doesn't mean you didn't submit to a pregnancy. You were still pregnant and the treatment alone is enough to cause real physical tension to your body. You do need recovery time.

Exhaustion is one thing that many women find they face the most, especially if they had surgery or a D&C. Anesthesia can make you very tired for at least a day and sometimes longer. It can also make you sick to your stomach if you had any kind of reaction to it. Plan on spending at least a day just relaxing and taking it easy. If you have any other children at home, consider asking someone for help with them. Be gentle and kind with yourself. This is the time to slip into bed, watch a movie, and be easy on your stomach.

If you live alone then you might want to ask someone to come and stay with you, just so that you don't have to be by yourself for the night. Once the anesthesia wears off you should be fine, but you might be a little sore and dizzy so you might need help getting to and from the bathroom and kitchen.

If you had major surgery, such as a hysterectomy, then you'll need to follow your doctor's orders and you'll be spending several days in the hospital. This is a major surgery and you won't be moving around like you are used to for a at least a couple of days - although they'll want you to get up and move after the first day so that you don't get blood clots.

Tips to help in your recovery

Follow all doctors' instructions and don't overdo it. Although it might feel as though you are feeling better sooner than you thought you would, if you do something too soon, you might land yourself back in the hospital.

People will probably volunteer to help. Let them. Accept offers when it comes to bringing you dinner, cleaning your house, watering your plants, feeding your cats, or even just bringing in your mail.

Don't be afraid to excuse yourself. If you don't feel like entertaining visitors, then just politely excuse yourself. People will understand.

Take all of your medication as per the directions. Don't skip any doses. Especially when it comes to pain medication (for surgery) and medication for depression, it is important to stay on top of these. They only work if you take them as directed. Make a schedule if you need to and then hand the meds over to someone you trust, like your partner or parent, and have that person disperse them to you.

Stay down. If you live in a house with two floors then try to sleep on the bottom floor for a week, at least, so that you don't have to use the stairs.

Go to the store. Invest in some sanitary pads to help soak up the bleeding. You'll also want some tight fitting underwear to help hold the pads in place. You'll really only need to wear these for a couple of days if you had a D&C, although if you have a hysterectomy you might need them longer.

Drink lots of fluids. It is important to stay hydrated. Not only will fluids help keep the toxins flushed out of your system, but many of the pain medications can cause constipation and the fluids will help prevent this.

Try relaxing. Meditating and other relaxation exercises can help you sleep better at night and help curb anxiety. Sleep is always a good thing, so is less anxiety.

Resuming physical activity after treatment

After surgery, rest is important. Although a D&C is an outpatient procedure, you might still feel some cramping and slight pain for a few days. A hysterectomy will require a significantly longer recovery period. Many women report feeling nauseated and exhausted after receiving chemotherapy treatments.

Even though you do need to get your rest, and rest will be a big part of your healing, there will come a point where it is important to start being active again. Some patients are surprised that their doctors and nurses have them up walking around within 24 hours of a major surgery, like a hysterectomy. A little bit of exercise, even a small walk around the room, will help prevent such complications as blood clots and bed sores. Later on, going outside for even 15 minutes a day without sunscreen and sunglasses can give you a healthy dose of vitamin D, which has been shown to reduce the symptoms of depression and anxiety.

There are some activities that might be limited at first, depending on your treatment. If you had a D&C then your doctor might recommend that you abstain from sexual intercourse for around 2 weeks, or at least until your bleeding has stopped. (Before the bleeding has stopped, the cervix can still be open and this can increase the chance of infection.)

If you had a hysterectomy then your doctor might suggest that you wait until your six week follow up before intercourse. Some women don't notice a difference in intercourse once they begin having it again, while others experience some dryness. This might mean that you need to use a water-based lubricant. A hysterectomy doesn't mean that you won't be able to achieve an orgasm since you'll still have your clitoris and labia.

Your doctor will probably suggest that you do pelvic floor exercises to aid in your physical recovery. These exercises, also called Kegel exercises, can also tone up your vaginal muscles and even improve sexual feeling. The pelvic floor muscles hold up the bladder and bowels and offer you control during urination. These are the muscles that you would use if you suddenly needed to halt your flow of urine.

To strengthen these, find a comfortable place to sit and squeeze the muscles 10-15 times in a row. It is important that you don't hold your breath or tighten your stomach or thigh muscles at the same time. In time, you should try to hold each squeeze for several seconds before releasing them. Make sure you rest in between. By doing these exercises on a daily basis after a surgery such as a hysterectomy, or a pregnancy, sensitivity during intercourse should improve.

Whether you've had a hysterectomy or a D&C, it is important that you listen to your doctor's advice about driving. After a D&C, don't drive or operate heavy machinery for 24 hours since anesthesia will still be in your system. If you are sent home with any pain medications then you might also be advised not to drive or operate machinery while on them. After a hysterectomy, you'll be in the hospital for at least the first 24 hours but after you are released you won't be able to drive for up to 6-8 weeks, depending on your doctors advice.

Your doctor might also give you advice about lifting. After a D&C, you shouldn't try to lift anything over 8 pounds for about 24 hours. After that, you should use caution. After a hysterectomy, your doctor might tell you not to lift anything over 20 pounds, or anything heavier than a gallon of milk, until you have your 6 week follow up. You must give your abdominal muscles time to heal and close back together. Bending and stretching should also be avoided for several weeks until those muscles have had the chance to heal, too. If you feel like you are doing something that's too much, then you probably are.

Women going through chemotherapy are generally not put on any physical restrictions, but the exhaustion can often make them feel limited on their own. Some women do not report feeling overly tired at all, while others feel exhausted after performing simple activities. Sometimes, the feeling of being on Methotrexate is described as "flu like" and it can be difficult to resume normal activities, such as work. Generally speaking, as your body gets used to it the tiredness does usually wear off and it is easier to go about your day and get things done.

Chapter 9: Conceiving Again

The good news is that even after experiencing a molar pregnancy you can still get pregnant again after most treatments (a hysterectomy notwithstanding, of course). It is still possible to become pregnant even if you've had chemotherapy. Your medical team should talk to you about this and what your best options are. After experiencing a molar pregnancy, 98% of women do go on to have normal pregnancies that result in live births. If you had a molar pregnancy without complications, your risk of having another molar pregnancy is about 1-2%.

How soon to conceive after GTD really depends on the kind of treatment you have had. Of course, most women want to start trying to conceive (TTC) right away.

In the past, it wasn't usually suggested that you try conceiving again before 6 months because if you were to become pregnant sooner it would be difficult to monitor your hCG levels and know whether or not your tumor was completely gone. This could be dangerous to both you and your new baby. It is particularly important to monitor your hCG levels in the first few months after treatment since that's when it is most likely to return.

If you simply had a D&C and your hCG levels have been regular for 3 months then your doctor will normally let you go ahead and start trying, as long as your hCG levels are normal. After the mole has been removed, hCG tests should be carried out every week until negative (<5) for three consecutive weeks, then every month for three consecutive months. If they remain negative then it should be safe to try and conceive.

If your treatment included chemotherapy then it is normally suggested that you wait at least a year before TTC. This will not only ensure that your hCG levels are normal again but that all of the medications are out of your system.

One of the biggest problems with TTC too soon, other than the chance that the mole could relapse, is that it can be difficult to know early on whether or not you have a viable pregnancy or if it is simply the mole returning when you are having the early blood work drawn. Since the embryo can't generally be seen on the ultrasound until 7-8 weeks, this can make the first trimester very stressful in a subsequent pregnancy that's already going to be very emotional.

If your hCG levels start out negative then at least you have a better chance of them increasing at a "normal" pregnancy rate, rather than giving a false increase and showing an abnormally high elevation in your first few blood tests.

At the very least, consider waiting 3 cycles before trying again and ensure that your levels are negative. When to try to conceive is really a choice that you and your partner have to make together and your doctor should be able to offer you advice on the matter.

Boosting your fertility

Once you are ready to start trying, you are going to want to ensure that your body is extra healthy and your fertility at an all time high so that you conceive as soon as possible. There are many different ways that you can boost your fertility, simply by making some changes and addressing your diet and lifestyle.

In the following section, we'll go over some tips that will help your mind and body prepare for the challenges (and fun) of conceiving again.

Of course, you don't have to try all of these, but they might give you some ideas to jumpstart your action plan and encourage you on your road to success.

Intercourse timing

It might be difficult having a healthy sex life even after you've recovered from your molar pregnancy. Some women find that grief actually enhances their desire while, for others, their desire wanes. If you are TTC, however, it is important to try and have fun with your sex life and not make it too mechanical, only having sexual intercourse on days that you are fertile. Of course this is often easier said than done. Your hormonal changes might lead you to experience a loss of your libido. Conversely, the idea of having another baby may make you feel like being more active.

Although you want to have intercourse on days that you are most fertile, aim for regular intercourse, even on the days when you are not ovulating. For your best chances of getting pregnant, try to have sex at least 3 times per week. That way you'll be sure to land on at least one of the days that you are fertile. The chances of conception increase from 15% for those engaging in intercourse once a week to 50% for those doing it 3-4 times per week.

Knowing your fertility symptoms can help you know when the best times for sexual intercourse are. Some of the signs include pain with ovulation (similar to period cramps), breast tenderness, light discharge, and mood swings. Increased cervical mucus, discharged from the vagina, is often the easiest sign to track.

Keep track of your cycles

Keeping track of your menstrual cycles is very important if you want to try to conceive again, no matter when that time may come.

It can be difficult to predict when your next cycle will start, especially if you've had chemo treatments, but it can be just as hard to predict it even if you've had a D&C. Your cycle may be delayed by weeks or even months after your hCG levels return to 0.

By tracking your cycles you'll have a better idea of when you are ovulating. You can also purchase an inexpensive ovulation kit from the drugstore, which can show you when your hormone levels are at their highest, giving you a good indication of the optimal time to conceive.

You can start by documenting your fertility signs and keeping track of your temperature changes. Some women keep a chart. On your chart you can record the length of the cycle, any positive ovulation tests, length of menstruation, any kind of spotting, or any other pertinent information.

Keeping this information handy may be helpful for diagnostic purposes or pregnancy dating when you do finally conceive. If you have trouble keeping it together yourself, there are several websites that can help you keep it documented and these have the added benefit of online forums which can give you support. Two websites that can be helpful when it comes to tracking your ovulation include:

> americanpregnancy.org
>
> and
>
> www.babycentre.co.uk

Go digital. These days, there are apps such as Fertility Friend and Period Diary that can be downloaded onto your phone or tablet, many of which are free. These can let you figure out when you are fertile and when your last menstrual cycle was.

Lifestyle watches. For extra help, there are now gadgets that can take some of the guesswork out of it for you. These "ovulation watches" detect changes in your chemical composition while you sleep. They're basically little computers that figure out if you are fertile by using a biosensor that detects chloride-ion levels from your skin through sweat. When you wake up in the morning, you just have to look at the watch to see if you are ovulating. Most watches can give you a 5-6 day fertility span, which is better than most urine tests which only give you a small window of opportunity - usually less than 36 hours. There are several out on the market but the OVWatch is the most popular and can be found at www.ovwatch.com.

Your mental health

Your emotions can rise and fall after experiencing a molar pregnancy. This can wreak havoc on your relationship. If you have a good support system, however, it can make things a little easier. A good support system can help alleviate the stress in your life. Getting support from other people in online forums or support groups can give you the advice and reassurance you need to lower your stress levels and make you more relaxed. Women naturally tend to conceive faster when they have less anxiety and are feeling more relaxed.

Stress can actually increase levels of cortisol, which is sometimes called the "stress hormone." If your body produces too much cortisol it can negatively affect the reproductive system. Stress can also have adverse affects on your relationship and make intercourse and intimacy in general more challenging.

Try to find something to help conquer the emotional anxiety that you are sure to encounter along the way. Things that may help include massage or acupuncture, exercise, writing down your feelings, talking to your partner or a professional and spending time outdoors.

Vitamin D. As previously mentioned, getting outside can be good for your mental health. However, it can also boost your fertility. Sunlight can actually increase fertility in both sexes by boosting levels of vitamin D. A study by the Medical University of Graz in Austria discovered that vitamin D increases the levels of the female sex hormones progesterone and estrogen. This can regulate menstrual cycles, thus making conception more likely. You don't have to spend a lot of time in the sunlight to get the benefits of vitamin D. 15 minutes a day without sunscreen or sunglasses is enough for most people – though of course less time is advisable in strong sunlight or if you burn easily. There are also some really great vitamin D supplements on the market.

Fewer chemicals

Parabens are a common toxin that can be found in many different personal care products, such as shampoos and lotions. They are preservatives and so can keep products from spoiling. However, when the body absorbs parabens, they can imitate estrogen. As a result, there is some concern that it might be dangerous to the reproductive system and hamper fertility.

The chemicals themselves are becoming more worrisome. In 2004, the UK Environment Agency conducted a survey on water pollution. The study discovered that a third of the male fish in the rivers that were studied had started growing female genitals; something they believe is the consequence of a buildup of "endocrine disrupters" in the environment. These same endocrine disruptors are the ones that are normally found in such things as food packaging and shampoo.

The European Union allows parabens in cosmetic products, but they have a limit as to the amount that can be added to the products. The Cosmetic Ingredient Review (CIR) evaluates ingredients for safety in the US. Although it recommends the same maximum concentration of parabens as the EU, this is a safety guideline for manufacturers and isn't a law.

When you are buying your personal care products, consider looking for those that are organic paraben-free or perhaps make your own at home.

Two companies that make good products that fit these guidelines are:

Jason   www.jason-personalcare.com

and Green People (they deliver worldwide)
www.greenpeople.co.uk

Diet

It is important to eat a healthy diet, even before you start trying to conceive again, but especially while you are pregnant.

A lot of doctors think a healthy diet can boost fertility, especially if you are suffering from certain ovulation issues such as ovulatory dysfunction or sub clinical PCOS (polycystic ovary syndrome).

Tips for a healthy diet include:

Protein. It is important to include protein in a healthy diet, though a lot of Americans rely too much on chicken, beef, and pork for it. The authorities at Harvard Medical School recommend replacing a serving of meat every day with protein such as tofu, beans, peas, or nuts as this can boost fertility.

Fresh fruits. Most fresh fruits are considered very healthy though try not to eat too much as they do still contain sugar. Those that contain vitamin B6, like bananas, can help regulate hormones. A B6 deficiency has been linked to poor sperm quality and irregular cycles. Berries are particularly good for fertility as they contain anti-oxidants which may help with egg quality and strawberries also contain folic acid.

Hydration. It is important to stay hydrated and drink plenty of water. Water helps create a strong supply of blood to the uterus' lining. In addition, staying hydrated will ensure that your cervical mucus, which helps the sperm to the egg, is fast moving.

Fiber. Fiber can help regulate blood sugar levels, which can reduce fertility issues and promote healthy hormonal balance. High fiber foods include dark leafy greens, fruits, vegetables, beans, and whole grains - bread where you can actually see the bits of grains in there.

Calcium. Eat plenty of milk, cheese, ice cream, yogurt, etc. A Harvard University study discovered that women who eat at least one serving of full-fat dairy every day can reduce their risk of infertility by more than 25%. Dairy can also encourage the ovaries to work more efficiently.

Iron. Iron is important in your overall health but a deficiency can also specifically impact fertility. Women who suffer from anemia may have lack of ovulation and poor egg health. This can hinder pregnancy at a rate that is 60% higher than those who are not anemic. Sources of iron include navy beans, tofu, lentils, kidney beans, molasses, spinach, and raw pumpkin seeds.

Colorful vegetables. Colorful vegetables offer a lot of vitamins and minerals and contain phytochemicals and antioxidants, which destroy free radicals and toxins. Free radicals can cause harm to the reproductive system, including sperm count. Some of the best vegetables are the ones that are brightly colored, such as red peppers and spinach. It is suggested that you try to eat at least 5 portions of brightly colored vegetables a day for optimum fertility.

Alkaline foods. Alkaline foods can determine your internal pH balance, which can affect your fertility. Most American diets are acid-forming since they contain a lot of meats, sugar, white flour, pastas, trans-fats, and dairy. Those who have highly stressful lives also tend to have acidity, too, since stress can affect the pH balance.

In an acidic environment, micro-organisms like yeast and other unhealthy bacteria can thrive. Some of these hinder the absorption of the essential vitamins and minerals that are in charge of the hormonal balance responsible for healthy reproduction and fertility. A very acidic environment can cause many fertility concerns such as vaginal infections, menstrual irregularities, urinary tract infections, prostatitis, infertility, and impotence.

Sperm prefer an alkaline environment and an alkaline diet can improve the quality of cervical mucus making it more sperm friendly. Foods to consume include papaya, spinach, kale, other leafy green vegetables, avocado, red peppers, wheatgrass, lemon-infused water, nuts, peas, sweet potatoes and olive oil. These will help create a more alkaline environment, which can naturally boost fertility.

It is also possible to invest in water cartridges or a water filter jug which will help make your tap water alkaline. Biocera is a good company to investigate if you are interested in this http://www.biocera.com.

Avoid acidic foods. Acidic foods, such as most processed foods, alcohol, and coffee can make your cervical mucus hostile to sperm.

Supplements

Supplements can be very helpful in boosting fertility and re-balancing your hormones, as well as improving you and your partner's general health.

Some vitamins and minerals can increase the likelihood of conception and implantation. Certain supplements can help get rid of any nutritional deficiencies and improve sperm production and mobility so that you can increase your chances of conceiving. The following is a short list of some of the most popular supplements. At the end of the book, you'll find links where some of these can be purchased.

Take a multi-vitamin. A study at the Royal Free Hospital in London found that taking a daily prenatal vitamin could more than double the chances of conception. Start taking vitamins for a few months before you begin trying to conceive. Most prenatal vitamin brands will include folic acid and it is never too soon to start taking it. Folic acid has been shown to decrease the chance of neural tube defects, including spina bifida.

Essential fatty acids (EFAs). EFAs such as omega-3s from fish and fish oil supplements have many health benefits. These include regulating your cycle, promoting blood flow to the uterus, supporting the opening of the follicle to release the egg and increasing cervical mucus.

Royal Jelly. Royal jelly is a substance that comes from the glands of worker bees and carries a lot of nutrients including vitamins D and E, amino acids, lipids, iron, calcium, and protein. Consuming it regularly might help balance hormones and offer support to the endocrine system. In 2007, a Japanese study determined that Royal Jelly can mimic the hormone estrogen. This might be helpful for those women who have lower levels of this hormone since estrogen is very important for a healthy menstrual cycle. Royal Jelly might also be helpful in increasing the libido, boosting the immune system, supporting egg health, and reducing inflammation.

Bee Propolis. Another natural supplement, this is a mixture of leaves, tree sap, tree buds, and additional botanical sources that the bees make in order to fasten up the small openings in their hives.

Bee propolis might be especially beneficial to those women who have any kind of scar tissue, either left over from surgery or from a medical condition. A study in *Fertility and Sterility* in 2003 showed that almost a third of women with endometriosis-related infertility who took bee propolis for 9 months went on to achieve pregnancy compared to 20% in the placebo group.

Bee propolis may also contain immune-modulating properties which could be valuable for fertility issues that are auto-immune related. Sometimes, a woman can be allergic to sperm due to certain antibodies in her system. Bee propolis might be able to protect against this.

However, if you are allergic to bees then bee products are not going to be an option for you.

Green powders. Green powders, such as FertiliGreens or Pure Synergy, may help support egg health. These powders, which are taken daily (usually mixed with a smoothie, water or juice), contain proteins, minerals, and antioxidants, which offer many health benefits and can alkalize the body.

L-Arginine. L-Arginine is a supplement that contains an essential amino acid. This is beneficial in supporting healthy circulation to the reproductive system for both genders. For women it can encourage blood flow to the ovaries and uterus and help stimulate cervical mucus production. In men it can encourage a healthy libido.

Fertility Blend. Researchers at Stanford University studied Fertility Blend, an herbal supplement, to see if it would help women who were having difficulty conceiving. Chasteberry is included in the supplement and it is thought that it might have an effect on hormonal imbalance and ovulation. In addition, the supplement contains green tea extract and L-arginine.

The study was published in 2004 in the *Journal of Reproductive Medicine*. Researchers found that a third of the women who took the supplement were pregnant after five months. However, none of the women who had taken the placebo had conceived.

The way you eat

Sometimes, it is not so much what you are eating as it is how you are eating it. Making simple lifestyle changes to how you approach your meals might give your fertility a boost. Here's how…

Eat at home. You might find that eating at home more often is valuable to your fertility. You have more control over your diet when you eat at home than when you eat out. In addition, eating home cooked meals that are made from scratch, rather than relying on pre-packaged meals, means that your body is not exposed to as many harmful chemicals and toxins such as additives and preservatives, which could hamper fertility.

Cook on the stove. If you do have any pre-packaged foods, then take them out of the plastic containers they came in and fix them in a metal or cast iron pot. When food is heated up in plastic containers, the containers have been known to release toxic chemicals, which could harm fertility.

Forgo the plastic bottles. Try to refrain from drinking out of plastic. If you do use plastic bottles, try to find some that are BPA (bisphenol-a) free. BPA, which is often used in hard plastic containers such as water bottles, has been known to cause a higher risk of diabetes, some forms of cancers, reduced fertility, and even birth defects (Neimark 2008).

Juicing. Fruits are good for you for many different reasons. However, fruit juices are another story. Most juices that you buy in the store like orange contain a huge amount sugar, some contain as much as soft drinks. An 8 oz. apple juice can have as much as 29 grams of sugar. This can cause blood sugar spikes and negatively affect your immune system. Rather than buying bottled juice, invest in a juicer and make your own at home.

When you invest in a juicer, you are getting the nutrients you need from the food without the added ingredients. You can make a juice from many vegetables and make it more palatable by adding half an apple or some berries. Plus, you can add many of the supplement powders to the juice you make which helps make them more digestible. Not only can the nutrients from the vegetables and fruit help boost fertility, but they can also help aid in your overall recovery, too, since a healthy diet can strengthen the immune system and encourage healing.

Juicers can be bought relatively inexpensively these days. Although you can certainly pay hundreds of dollars (or pounds) for one, it is also possible to purchase a good juicer for less than $60 or £40 sterling.

In the United States, Hamilton Beach, CuisinArt, and Black & Decker all make juicers for less than $60, with CuisinArt's Pulp Control Citrus Juicer coming in at a low $29.99.

In the UK, the Bistro (sold by Bodum) gets good reviews and is mid-priced at £52.90. Cuisinart offers a unit for £150 that's easy to clean and has an adjustable sprout while Kenwood, at Tesco, is an affordable £29.97 and is dishwasher safe. At the end, you can find links to some of the juicers and where to purchase them.

When you use a juicer to make your own juice, you need to drink it almost immediately. You can't save it for very long. One of the perks of fresh juice is that it doesn't have any additives or preservatives in it. Of course, this also means that it won't have a long shelf life. Fixing yourself a glass of fresh vegetable juice is a great healthy way to start off the morning, though, or have a quick snack in the afternoon and now you won't have to worry about any chemicals that might be lurking in it.

Blood sugar. Keep your blood sugar levels regulated. Try to avoid any spikes, highs or lows. This might mean keeping a light healthy snack on you, such as a gluten-free oat biscuit, so that you never get too hungry. Some authorities believe that a diet that contains a lot of refined carbohydrates, such as white bread and pasta, can affect conception. Refined carbs can cause blood sugar to spike and this can lead to an insulin surge, which might damage fertility.

Alternative therapies

Although western medicine has come a long way, there are some proven ways of boosting fertility that rely on methods that have been successfully used for thousands of years. These "alternative therapies" might not be for everyone, but many of them offer stress-reducing effects and can be good for your mental health, as well as your reproductive system.

Reflexology. Not only is reflexology a good way to help you relax, it can also help boost fertility. It works in a variety of ways, but mostly by helping the different organs and systems in your body that support the reproductive system function at their best. It can help boost fertility by doing the following:

- Working the pituitary gland, which produces a lot of the hormones that regulate the menstrual cycle.

- Helping improve the thyroid's function. Both hypo- and hyperthyroidism can negatively impact fertility.

- Stimulate the ovaries to help them produce eggs and estrogen.

- Help increase blood flow to the uterus.

Acupuncture. Acupuncture is another method of healing that's been used as a form of medicine for 2,500 years. It has been known to boost fertility and it is often used to help IVF patients. It is an ancient Chinese medicine treatment that uses the deliberate placement of small needles in a pattern on the body. The needles stimulate "energy points" that are thought to control your physical, spiritual, mental, and emotional equilibrium. Acupuncture can help by addressing issues that might affect fertility such as hypothyroidism or hyperthyroidism. Since it can help your body operate more efficiently, this can let more contemporary treatments, such as IVF, work more effectively as well.

Acupuncture can help stimulate the growth and later release of eggs and lead to more successful implantations, too. In a German study conducted in 2002 and published in *Fertility and Sterility* it was discovered that women only needed to have two 25-minute sessions (one before IVF implantation and one following) to see a significant boost in pregnancies. In fact, of the 160 women in the study, 42% who received acupuncture conceived in comparison to the 26% of those who did not.

Detox. Many women experience gastrointestinal issues, especially if they have other underlying problems such as endometriosis. We are exposed to toxins from our environment every day, from the preservatives in our food, to stress and lifestyle choices which can result in hormonal imbalance, premature ageing, allergies, food intolerance, obesity, and infertility. A detox can help eliminate toxic substances and strengthen the body's ability to detoxify naturally. It can also improve the circulation of blood to the ovaries, uterus, and the pituitary gland. A detox might also help regulate the menstrual cycle, improve implantation, and help remove any heavy metal deposits from the uterus, fallopian tubes and other reproductive organs that might be contributing to infertility.

There are two ways of going about a detox: doing one all at once or doing a gradual detox. In a sudden detox, you fast and eliminate food almost completely (most detoxes call for juices and/or broths) over a period of days. In a gradual detox, you would most likely get tested for food intolerances and then start eliminating those foods from your diet. Either way, your body will be able to eliminate the things that are harmful to it and that it doesn't need, such as heavy metals.

Of course a detox can be quite an undertaking and it is recommend that you seek the advice of a health professional before attempting one. In addition, if you suspect that you might already be pregnant, or there's a chance that you are, then you should avoid doing a detox.

Chinese herbs. Chinese medicine has been used to boost fertility in men and women for a long time. It centers on creating holistic balance, with the aim being to determine which organ systems are out of balance and then to treat that. Although western medicine treats the disease, Chinese medicine treats the person. If you go to a Chinese herbalist for help, they will treat you like you would be treated at a regular doctor's office. You'll be asked about your symptoms and then the herbalist will try to determine which organ systems are out of balance. A herbal formula will then be customized for you.

In cases of infertility, Chinese medicine has been used to help regulate menstrual cycles, regulate hormone levels, and boost healthy sperm count. There haven't been many studies conducted on infertility and Chinese medicine but a few have shown success rates. For instance, in a study at a university in Tel Aviv, a group of women who were going through intrauterine insemination was dived into two groups. One group submitted to acupuncture and took traditional Chinese medicine as part of their treatment, while the others didn't. Those taking the Chinese herbs had a 65.5% conception rate while the others had only a 39.4% success rate. In the UK, a study of Chinese herbal medicine found that over a series of different trials there was a 3.5 times greater chance of conceiving while using traditional Chinese medicine.

You do need to be aware, however, that Chinese herbs, like Western medicine, can cause side effects. You should always see a professional and check if there are any known side effects before starting any treatment.

Meditation/positive visualization. Meditating and using creative visualization can be a good way to help encourage the reality you want to manifest. Some top athletes use visualization to help them before a big game, since they believe that seeing themselves actually make the basket or touchdown (or goal) in their minds will help them do it during the actual event.

Meditation can be a wonderful way of relaxing your body and your mind, but some people believe that positive visualization can help you create the energy around you that you need in order to bring forth the things you desire into your life. While you are meditating, try to focus on visualizing yourself being pregnant. Visualize the conception, the embryo, the growing fetus, the baby and the different stages of the pregnancy and hopefully this will make you feel both relaxed and positive.

Massage. Relaxing and decreasing your anxiety can help boost fertility and few methods are as effective as helping you relax as a good massage. A study published in a 2004 issue of the *International Journal of Neurosciences* found that massage considerably reduces stress. In just a 10 minute treatment, the subjects experienced a decrease in anxiety. A stomach massage during ovulation might help boost fertility by helping position the uterus in the optimal position and remove blockages that might exist in the fallopian tubes. In an article entitled "Gynecologists Investigate Massage As Infertility Treatment" on Personal MD, early research showed a remarkable reversal in 75% of infertility cases that involved tubal blockages (Gynecologists Investigate Massage as Infertility Treatment, 2000).

Additional benefits of a fertility massage can include:

* Assisting in the breakdown of adhesions and scar tissue
* Improving digestion
* Increasing blood flow to the reproductive organs
* Reducing inflammation that can be caused by ovarian cysts or uterine fibroids

Feng shui. Some people believe that not only should you focus on your body when you are trying to conceive, but you should also focus on your home. The ancient art of feng shui believes that infertility can be partly attributed to energy, called chi, that is blocked or inactive. Feng shui tries to balance the energy of a room (or place in general) to offer a person the optimal health while in that space.

When your body and mind is in harmony then your energy flows like it is supposed to. However, if something is "off" within the environment and doesn't follow the core of feng shui principles then the energy can become stagnant. Those who follow the principles of feng shui believe this might lead to infertility in the same way it can cause headaches or tiredness.

You can focus on balancing the energy in your bedroom since that's probably where the conception will take place. When trying to conceive, you want to balance your female energy (yin) and male energy (yang). You can do this by using calming colors and decorations in your bedroom to create a beautiful room. Colors such as pink, gold, and tan can promote both sexual intimacy and harmony. On the other hand, in keeping with feng shui, you want to keep the fresh flowers and floral pillows out since flowers are considered the male expression of a plant and this might be considered competition with your partner's yang and throw off the balance.

You can also eliminate TVs or computers from your bedroom. You want your bedroom to be considered a place of relaxation, sleep and intimacy and not used for another purpose, such as watching television or working. Lastly, even the way you sleep can affect feng shui. According to these principles, a woman should lay on the right side and the man on the left side of the bed since this is meant to balance the energy of the couple.

Yoga. Yoga isn't just a workout; it is a form of meditation that for many is relaxing. Yoga can also help boost fertility by not only offering a more peaceful atmosphere within the body but key yoga poses can help support and strengthen the endocrine and reproductive systems. The endocrine system is important for good hormonal balance. Yoga can also increase circulation to your reproductive system, support a healthy immune system, and possibly help remove blockages that are present in the reproductive areas.

If you've never tried yoga before then you might want to go with a beginner's class, or a gentle style such as Kripalu or basic Hatha. Other styles such as Ashtanga or Bikram can be more energetic and are usually more suitable for those who are more advanced.

You might find a yoga group or classes at a community center, local college or university, gym, YMCA, or fitness center. Some fitness centers allow you to pay by the class so that you don't have to buy an entire membership to the center.

Exercise

Exercising might not be fun for everyone but the better shape you are in before you get pregnant, the easier it will be to handle some of the challenges your body will face when you are pregnant. It can even boost fertility. If you are a little overweight then losing a few extra pounds before you conceive might be necessary. It is better to do this before you get pregnant because most doctors do not recommended that you try to lose weight while you are pregnant and dieting while pregnant is almost never recommended.

Extra body fat can actually cause an overproduction of certain hormones that can disturb ovulation. This can lead to irregular cycles and cycles in which you don't ovulate at all. If you are overweight, even losing just 5% of your body weight can boost chances of conceiving by about a fifth. Conversely, being underweight isn't healthy either. If you have too little body fat then your body may not produce enough hormones to ovulate every month. In this case, gaining as few as 5 pounds (which can be done as muscle through exercise) might be enough to help trigger your cycle to becoming regular.

You don't have to go into weight lifting or run a marathon, but exercising even 20 minutes a day, 3 times per week can help. Get a friend involved for support and encouragement and try going for a walk around the neighborhood, ride your bike up and down the road, pop in an exercise tape, or join a zumba group in town. Swimming is very easy on the joints if you suffer from something such as fibromyalgia or arthritis and it is an excellent workout for just about anyone. Many health centers offer water aerobic classes.

Unless you are used to exercising heavily, it is best not to take this up during your pregnancy. This is something you should talk to your doctor about.

Things to avoid

Along with adding certain things to your lifestyle in order to boost fertility, sometimes it is necessary to avoid or eliminate other things. The following is a list of things that you should at least try to cut back on, if you can't stay away completely.

Smoking. Of course, you should avoid smoking and taking recreational drugs while you are pregnant, but you should also try to avoid smoking when you are trying to conceive as well. Women who smoke have a 30% lower fertility rate than those who don't. Smoking can also inhibit implantation.

Alcohol. Too much alcohol has been found to harm both ovulation and sperm production. A Swedish study discovered that women who drank two alcoholic beverages a day decreased their fertility by nearly 60%.

Caffeine. Some studies show that too much caffeine could increase the chance of miscarriage, but someone women are unable to cut back on their caffeine intake due to other health problems, such as migraines, so this is something that you'll have to consider. Caffeine could diminish the activity of the fallopian tube muscles. These are important since they transport the eggs from the ovaries.

Limit pain pills. Try to use natural forms of pain relief when possible. Some pain pills, like paracetamol and ibuprofen, might affect conception if you take them around the time you are ovulating. It is possible that they could hold back prostaglandins, the hormones that help release the eggs into the fallopian tube. Instead of relying on pain pills, try to use light exercise, stretching, and ice or heat on the painful areas.

Fat-Free Foods. Foods that are listed as "fat free" can actually be damaging when you are trying to conceive. These are more likely to be highly processed and high in sugar.

Exposure to pesticides. Agricultural pesticides might damage both men and women's fertility. Regular exposure to some toxins, such as those used in printing and dry cleaning businesses, can also negatively affect a woman's fertility. Avoid your exposure to these when you can.

Foods that can contain listeria. Listeria is a dangerous bacterium that can be discovered in things such as soft cheeses and ready-to-eat meats. It can also be found in unpasteurized dairy products. Women who are trying to conceive should be cautious since the infection caused by listeria can cause a miscarriage early in the first trimester, often before the woman knew she was even pregnant. To reduce the risk of this bacteria growth on leftovers, set your refrigerator's temperature to 40ºF (4ºC) or below. Throw away any food that's been left out at room temperature for more than two hours. Avoid: soft cheese made from raw milk, raw sushi, refrigerated smoked seafood, refrigerated pâté or meat spreads, and other unpasteurized dairy products.

Some fish. Most fish is considered very healthy, especially fish that contain omega-33, but some fish have high mercury content and this can be dangerous to a growing fetus. Since mercury can build up in the body and stay for as long as a year, avoiding fish that's high in mercury such as swordfish, tilefish, and shark is recommended. Instead of these fish, try eating fish that contain healthy fats such as salmon.

Your partner's fertility

Although the pregnancy is going to take place in your body, you also have to be concerned with your partner's sperm health. In order to conceive, he must have healthy sperm, which means his sperm count and the quality of his sperm may need to be boosted.

Many of the fertility problems that affect couples are due to an issue with the sperm. Your partner can help boost his sperm count and quality by focusing on having a healthy diet, cutting back on alcohol and cigarettes, taking a multi-vitamin, and following some of the other tips below.

Diet

If your partner wants to boost his fertility, there are some dietary changes he can make in his life, too. The following have been helpful in increasing sperm count and leading to successful pregnancies.

Pumpkin seed: Pumpkin seeds contain phytosterols, protective compounds that can help shrink an enlarged prostate and improves testosterone production. The omega-3 fatty acids can also help improve blood flow to the penis.

Maca powder: Peruvians have used Maca to boost fertility for years. Studies have shown that in powder form it can boost sperm count. Maca powder can be found at many health food stores. It can also help boost female fertility.

Spinach: When you eat spinach with foods high in vitamin C to help with absorption, the folic-acid helps increase overall sperm health.

Multi-vitamin: Studies have found that men who took 5 mg of folic acid and 66 mg of zinc sulfate a day for 26 weeks had an almost 75% increase in sperm count. In addition, Vitamin C and selenium may also be helpful in increasing sperm count.

Vitamin E foods: Vitamin E can be found in foods such as spinach, sunflower seeds, olives, and dark leafy greens. Vitamin E can help improve sperm health and motility in men.

Zinc. A zinc deficiency can make sperm cluster together and lead to infertility. Good sources of zinc include oysters, dark chicken meat, extra-lean beef tenderloin, and baked beans.

Folic acid. Low levels of folic acid in men may lead to poor quality sperm. Nutritionists recommend 400 micrograms of folic acid per day. Sources of this B vitamin can come from leafy green vegetables, orange juice, legumes, and fortified breakfast cereals. However, some men might also want to consider taking a supplement if they feel like they might not be able to reach 400 micrograms through diet alone.

Orange juice. Once you start making your own fresh juice, your partner can start boosting his vitamin C. Vitamin C, found in orange juice, can help prevent sperm defects and boost motility.

Things to avoid

Overheating. The best sperm grows in a cool atmosphere. It has been shown that men who sit with laptops on their laps can experience reduced fertility rates. Your partner should also try to avoid taking any hot baths. Taking a cool shower instead of a hot bath can increase sperm production by as much as 5 times.

Tight underwear. For optimal sperm production, encourage your partner to wear loose fitting boxer shorts instead of tight underwear, which could decrease blood flow to their pelvic region.

Smoking. Not only should you quit smoking, your partner should quit as well. Men who smoke are 50% more likely to be impotent and have lower sperm counts. The quality of their sperm tends not to be as good, either.

Caffeine: Studies have shown that men who drink a quart of cola on a regular basis have 30% less sperm than men who do not.

Soy-based foods: Your partner should try to avoid soy. Soy-based foods and high-fructose corn syrup contain a mild estrogenic effect on the body. This is not good for sperm. High-fructose corn syrup causes insulin resistance and this can lower fertility.

Of course, a decrease in **alcohol** can also help increase your partner's sperm count.

An action plan to get you started

Now that you have some ideas to follow, you might want to create an action plan so you can use the down time after a molar pregnancy to get your fertility into the best shape.

The following is simply an example as the important thing is that you create a plan that is completely tailored to your specific needs, and goals. Some of the suggestions listed in this chapter may resonate with you, others just won't feel right for you personally. The important thing is that you use only those which appeal to you and that you feel instinctively could make a difference.

No-one could possibly hope or want to include all the suggestions listed and to try and do so would be counter-productive as it could leave you with little time for anything else! Just try and set yourself some achievable goals which will boost your fertility and empower you to feel more positive about the future.

Example Plan

Month 1

Start taking multi-vitamins, including folic acid.

Consider which if any supplements are right for you and start taking them.

Practice creative visualization.

Get at least 15 minutes of sunlight every day for vitamin D.

Begin a healthy eating plan and eliminate alcohol. Cut back on caffeine.

Get partner involved in healthy heating plan.

Eliminate as many products with harmful chemicals as possible, ie. parabens.

Start a light exercise regimen.

Consider a detox to kick start your fertility program.

Month 2

Continue taking fertility supplements: Royal Jelly, Maca powder, etc.

Continue creative visualization and meditation.

Start tracking menstrual cycle to chart ovulation and/or purchase ovulation kit from store and start urine tests.

Continue healthy diet, including more homemade meals.

Consider investing in a juicer and prepare lots of vegetable rich juices for both you and your partner.

Take time to relax and explore if reflexology, acupuncture or massage might help with this for you.

Consider a water filter which will help your body become more alkaline

Month 3

Continue with multi-vitamins.

Continue with fertility supplements.

Continue creative visualization and meditation.

Sign up for yoga course and/or continue light exercise.

Keep eating really healthily and ensure you include lots of bright coloured vegetables.

Make appt. with doctor for check-up to ensure everything looks good.

When your doctor confirms you are ready to start trying again, aim for intercourse at least 3 times per week.

Chapter 10: What to expect in a subsequent pregnancy

Some women want to try to conceive again right away. Others want to wait. Some women may feel so scarred by their molar pregnancy that they feel very nervous about attempting another pregnancy.

It might lessen your fears to know that a molar pregnancy does not mean you are going to have a baby in the future that's "damaged." The GTD does not place your unborn baby at risk for any irregular abnormalities - at least not at any greater risk than any other child is. Your odds are still extremely low.

In a study published in 2003 conducted at the Supraregional Trophoblastic Disease Unit in London, England found that 98% of women who went on to conceive after having a molar pregnancy removed weren't at any increased risk of other obstetric complications. A previous molar pregnancy therefore does *not* increase your risk for:

- Pre-term delivery
- Birth defects
- Stillbirth
- Other complications

There's no doubt about it, the subsequent pregnancy is going to be an emotional one. You shouldn't attempt conceiving again until you feel emotionally able to handle the roller-coaster ride that it is going to be. It won't be easy to face the uphill battle that you are going to face at almost every doctor's visit as you wait for blood test results and ultrasound scans as you listen for heartbeats and reassurance. Then, there will be more stress as you wonder whether or not your hCG levels are where they need to be.

Of course, all of this will be worth it if you want to have a baby.

The first trimester is generally the hardest. Once you get through it, and you can be assured that the pregnancy is a viable one, then the rest of the pregnancy is generally a little smoother.

Confronting the emotional fears is important. When you simply push them aside, they still exist and will continue to find their way back. They won't go away.

Some women find that even though they wanted to get pregnant again, they have trouble forming a connection with the present pregnancy and, instead, want the former pregnancy back. They feel guilty for their present pregnancy and "miss" the old one. It is important not to dismiss these feelings and to recognize them for what they are, fear and anxiety, and to deal with them instead of ignoring them.

It is important to try when both you and your partner are ready. Although you might be ready a lot sooner than your partner, you must take their feelings into consideration. Getting pregnant too soon might put a strain on your relationship and this could make for a very stressful pregnancy - something that isn't good for anyone. Being on the same page is valuable, even if that means waiting a few more months.

Since your pregnancy is almost certainly going to be considered a high risk one, you can almost guarantee that you are going to be getting more ultrasounds, or scans, than most people.

If you don't have a regular OBGYN or weren't happy with the one you had in your last pregnancy then find one you like before you get pregnant. "Audition" them if you must, although be aware that your health insurance might not pay for more than one visit. You need a supportive doctor who will take your concerns seriously and actually answer your questions and make you feel secure. After you conceive your OBGYN should see you promptly, perform all blood tests that monitor your pregnancy such like hCG or progesterone level testing, and screen you with an early ultrasound. Most women feel more comfortable getting this sorted out before they conceive so that they're not rushing around trying to find a good doctor they trust once they find out they're pregnant.

If you've had multiple molar pregnancies, consider working with a perinatologist. These doctors are board certified in perinatology which is the study and care of problem pregnancies. They can work with a team that includes an ultra-sonographer, specialized lab technicians, a geneticist and a nurse specialist. They'll conduct a thorough history and physical, review reports of previous exams and labs and determine if you needed additional testing.

The first scan will be the one that shows viability. This one will come in at about 7-8 weeks. It will look for an embryo, heart, or egg sac. Another scan might be done at week 11 or 12.

At around 18 or 20 weeks your doctor will do what's commonly referred to as the "anatomy" scan. This is the most exciting scan because it is the one that tells you the gender. It is possible to tell the gender as soon as 16 weeks, depending on how the baby is positioned, but it's usually done around 18 weeks. This scan is normally a long one and will take about 30 minutes. You should get quite a few shots of him or her.

An additional scan will be performed at around 32 weeks to check on the lungs on and heart and to make sure they're functioning the way they're supposed to be. Of course, if you are experiencing any symptoms in between those weeks that need to be checked out then your doctor might perform additional scans as well.

You might have increased anxiety during your pregnancy, which could make some of your pregnancy symptoms, such as nausea, worse. It is important to talk to your doctor about your fears and to feel comfortable with your medical team. If you don't feel comfortable with the healthcare you are getting then feel free to find someone else. After all, this is your body and your child you are receiving care for. Your doctor needs to be on the same page as you. The more comfortable you feel, the more relaxed you'll be and the more pleasant an experience your pregnancy will be.

Some women wonder when they should announce their subsequent pregnancy. In this day and age, with everyone announcing even trivial things via social media, many people are no longer waiting the traditional 12 weeks to announce their pregnancies anymore. However, if it makes you feel better to wait until you know for sure that it is a viable pregnancy then you might want to wait until you are well into your second trimester before you announce your next pregnancy. Of course, it is entirely up to you. Other women find that they want and need the support from their family and friends and that by announcing it early they get that support a lot sooner.

If you have trouble conceiving

If you try to conceive for 6 months and find that you still haven't, or that you are not having a menstrual cycle at all, then talk to your doctor. It is possible that you could have some tissue scarring in your uterus. An ultrasound can show whether or not you are shedding the lining in your uterus each month and this can help your doctor determine what steps to take.

It is important to note that most women will not have a menstrual cycle until their hCG levels have dropped down close to 0 and some women won't have one until several weeks after their D&C, usually at least 4 weeks.

A hysterosonogram can break up any scar tissue by using saline and help encourage a menstrual cycle, too. A hysteroscopy can also be done to remove some of the scar tissue as well. This is a small surgery that can be performed as an outpatient procedure.

Most women are able to conceive within 12 months of trying. According to statistics on http://www.babycentre.co.uk:

- 20% of fertile couples conceive within the first month of trying

- 70% conceive within 6 months of trying

- 85% conceive within one year

- 90% conceive within 18 months

- 95% conceive within two years

For women in the United States, the statistics on http://www.babycenter.com include the following:

- 30% conceive within the first month

- 59% conceive within 3 months

- 80% conceive within 6 months of trying

- 85% conceive within one year

If you haven't been able to conceive within a year, even after trying some of the fertility boosting tips previously mentioned, then you might want to discuss other options with your doctor. There are certain fertility enhancing drugs that are often prescribed for women who are having difficulty conceiving and these can be discussed with your doctor as well. It is therefore important to keep track of your cycle, as mentioned above, and discuss any concerns you have about conceiving with him or her.

Conclusion

There is no doubt about it, a molar pregnancy can be a very scary and heartbreaking ordeal. With such a large percentage of women going on to conceive again after experiencing a mole, however, there's no reason to think that it can't happen for you as well. From dietary changes to learning new techniques to help you relax, there are lots of ways to boost fertility and the trying part of conceiving can be half the fun!

If you choose not to move forward with a subsequent pregnancy then it is still important to keep up with any follow-up appointments you have with your doctor, especially for the first few months after your treatment. Molar pregnancies have an almost 100% cure rate and even if they become persistent or malignant the cure rate is still almost 100%, but it is essential to seek treatment when there are signs of the disease. By submitting to regular blood tests to check you hCG levels and listening to your own body to be aware of your symptoms you can feel confident in your prognosis.

In the future, there is hope that with more awareness and research one day there will be a prevention for molar pregnancies and this won't be a heartache that so many women have to needlessly suffer. In the meantime, it is important to keep being optimistic and feel confident that you are doing everything you can to ensure your own body and mind are as healthy as they can be and that, if you are trying to conceive, you are doing everything in your power to boost your chances of seeing that pregnancy sooner rather than later.

Glossary of Terms

Anemia: A condition in which an individual possesses fewer red blood cells, the cells that transport oxygen to bodily tissues, than they should. Anemia can also be considered an iron deficiency.

Beta qual: The blood test that discovers a pregnancy based on the blood's hCG levels. Although it detects the existence of elevated hCG, it doesn't give a precise amount.

Beta quant: The blood test that finds the precise amount of hCG levels in women who have gestational trophoblastic neoplasia. This test is used in the discovery of non-routine recognition of hCG. The "standard" levels of hCG are usually less than 5, though this can vary depending on the doctor.

Choriocarcinoma: This is the cancerous form of gestational trophoblastic neoplasia. Although it originally develops within the placental tissue it can metastasize and travel to other areas of the body. It treated aggressively; it is normally curable if it is caught early on.

Complete mole: A molar pregnancy that happens when the sperm fertilizes an empty egg sac. Although a baby isn't formed, placental tissue still develops and hCG is produced.

Dilation and curettage (D&C): A D&C is a minor procedure, usually outpatient, in which the cervix is stretched (dilated) enough to allow the lining of the uterus to be scraped with an instrument called a curette. This procedure is usually carried out after a miscarriage or an abortion in order to ensure that all tissue has been removed for safety and health concerns.

Ectopic pregnancy: In an ectopic pregnancy, the fertilized egg implants in the fallopian tube, ovary, or abdominal cavity instead of within the uterus.

Embryo: The developing offspring in terms of the pregnancy. Some doctors refer to the pregnancy as an embryo until the second trimester when it is then considered a fetus, although this terminology can vary.

Endometriosis: A condition in which the uterine lining grows on the outside of the uterus. It can grow on the uterus, ovaries, fallopian tubes, and even on the intestines and stomach.

Epithelioid trophoblastic tumors (ETT): A type of malignant tumor that is often found in the uterine cervix or lower uterine area.

Gestational trophoblastic disease (GTD): A group of conditions in which tumors can develop inside a uterus. The irregular tissues grow from what would ordinarily be the placenta. Rather than producing a viable embryo, in some cases there is an empty egg sac while in others there is some embryonic tissue but it is usually defective and the pregnancy is still not considered a viable one. The hydatidiform mole is the most common of these conditions and is also referred to as a molar pregnancy.

Gestational trophoblastic neoplasia (GTN): This is a general term for any condition in which potentially cancerous cells grow within the placental tissues. This can include both molar pregnancy and choriocarcinoma.

Human chorionic gonadotropin, hCG: A placenta-produced hormone that is detected by blood and urine pregnancy tests.

Hydatidiform mole: Another name for a molar pregnancy. An irregular growth that surrounds the embryo and generates the placenta. If a mole develops, the embryo is typically either missing or deceased. The mole is a group of cysts that look like a cluster of grapes can grow quite large. If not removed soon, they can spread into surrounding tissues and cause bleeding and other problems. They can develop into choriocarcinoma in rare instances.

Hyperemesis gravidarum: An often severe complication of pregnancy that can be characterized by constant nausea and vomiting which can lead to malnutrition and weight loss.

Molar pregnancy: A pregnancy in which a genetic issue occurs during fertilization and an abnormality and a mass forms in the uterus instead of a viable embryo.

Partial mole: A molar pregnancy that occurs when two sperm fertilize the same egg. An embryo is formed, but is usually extremely defective and abnormal and the pregnancy is not viable.

Placental-site trophoblastic tumors: A rare tumor that forms at the site where the placenta was attached to the uterus.

Preeclampsia: The development of high blood pressure and protein in the urine during pregnancy.

Subchorionic hematoma: Also called a subchorionic hemorrhage, this is when blood pools between the membranes of the placenta and the uterus and causes bleeding during pregnancy.

Salpingectomy: A surgery in which the fallopian tube is removed.

Theca lutein cysts: Fluid filled sacs that can form on the ovaries. These mostly occur when hCG levels are high and they can range from feeling uncomfortable to being very painful.

Ultrasound, abdominal: A noninvasive procedure in which sound waves are used to produce images of the inside of the stomach cavity. The reflected sound waves are received by instruments called *transducers*. These are small, hand-held devices that are slide back and forth across the abdomen to produce an image on a screen. To help assist in the movement, a lubricating gel is normally placed on the stomach.

Ultrasound, transvaginal: A form of ultrasound in which special probes are inserted into the vagina. These are often more helpful in gaining better images of the fetus and other uterine conditions in the early part of the pregnancy. A lubricating gel is normally applied to the unit to make insertion easier.

Additional Helpful Resources

There are a large number of sites which offer more information, support groups and vendors of products or other services. The following list is only a small percentage of those.

Inclusion in this list or in the text of this book does not indicate endorsement of the organisation or any products or vendors. Neither does absence from the list indicate lack of approval. Buyers should study any products carefully to ensure they meet their needs.

There will inevitably be changes to sites and addresses which are not possible to track in a publication like this. We are planning a website to accompany the book which we will update periodically to ensure the links are current and to allow us to expand the database. Please feel free to visit us at www.molarpregnancy.info.

Online forums

Sites which have molar pregnancy support threads:

Mumsnet: http://www.mumsnet.com/talk

BabyCentre (UK):   http://www.babycentre.co.uk

BabyCenter (US):   http://www.babycenter.com

My Molar Pregnancy Facebook Support Group:
        https://www.facebook.com/groups/315375955180318/

After My Molar Pregnancy (TTC) Facebook Support Group:
https://www.facebook.com/groups/319276728136446/

Silent Grief- online chat board for those who have lost
pregnancies and infants: http://www.silentgrief.com/

Help Her-Hyperemesis Education & Research
  An active online forum as well as extensive information
  and recent research: www.helpher.org

Hyster Sisters
  An active online forum and information site relating to
  hysterectomies: www.hystersisters.com

Charities

Hygeia Foundation- supporting the loss of a pregnancy or infant: hygeiafoundation.org

March of Dimes- Ectopic and Molar Pregnancy page:
www.marchofdimes.com/loss/ectopic-and-molar-pregnancy.aspx

Mary Stolfa Cancer Foundation:
marystolfacancerfoundation.org/GestationalTrophoblasticTumors.html

Cancer Research UK

A nonprofit organization, but it also has an information page on trophoblastic disease:

Angel Building, 407 St John Street, London EC1V 4AD

www.cancerreasearchuk.org

Information sites

Molar Pregnancy Support & Information

Forums, FAQs, and general information site related to molar pregnancies. The founder suffered from a molar pregnancy herself and shares her story. A section is set aside for members to share their stories as well:

www.molarpregnancy.co.uk

The NHS' Molar Pregnancy information site (UK):
www.nhs.uk/conditions/Molar-pregnancy/Pages/Introduction.aspx

My Molar Pregnancy: mymolarpregnancy.com

American Cancer Society which has a page on trophoblastic disease, including current research:

www.cancer.org

Baby Zone: Understanding Molar Pregnancy:
www.babyzone.com/pregnancy/pregnancy-complications/molar-pregnancy_78812

American Pregnancy Association: Molar Pregnancy:
americanpregnancy.org/pregnancycomplications/molarpregnancy.html

Medscape's informational page on Gestational trophoblastic neoplasia: emedicine.medscape.com/article/279116-overview

International Society for the Study of Trophoblastic
Diseases: www.isstd.org/isstd/home.html

National Cancer Institute (NCI): www.cancer.gov

Miscarriage Support-molar pregnancy (New Zealand):
www.miscarriagesupport.org.nz/molar.html

What is molar pregnancy You Tube video:
www.youtube.com/watch?v=LcZbuc8raOQ&feature=youtu.be

What is molar pregnancy You Tube video:
www.youtube.com/watch?v=bprrUG6i3pM&feature=youtu.be

Miscarriage Association

They have a booklet on molar pregnancy at:
www.miscarriageassociation.org.uk

American Congress of Obstetricians and Gynecologists
(ACOG): www.acog.org

The Ectopic Pregnancy Trust

An informational site about ectopic pregnancies:
www.ectopic.org.uk

Where to go for help

Charing Cross Hospital Trophoblast Disease Service (UK):
www.hmole-chorio.org.uk

Sheffield Trophoblastic Disease Centre (UK):
www.chorio.group.shef.ac.uk

Dana Farber Cancer Institute (US)

Information on Trophoblastic cancer and where to seek help, including treatment options:
www.dana-farber.org

The Cleveland Clinic (US):   my.clevelandclinic.org

HAND - Helping After Neonatal Death:
www.handonline.org

Memorial Sloan-Kettering Cancer Center (US):
www.mskcc.org/cancer-care/adult/gestational-trophoblastic-disease

Acupuncture

American Board of Medical Acupuncture:
www.dabma.org

Acupuncture Society of America, Inc:
www.acupuncturesociety.org

Acupuncture-Gateway to Chinese Medicine, Health, &
Wellness: www.acupuncture.com/

The Acupuncture Society:
www.acupuncturesociety.org.uk

The British Medical Acupuncture Society:
www.medical-acupuncture.co.uk

The British Acupuncture Council:
www.acupuncture.org.uk

Reflexology

Association of Reflexologists: www.apr.org.uk

Reflexology Association of America:
www.reflexology-usa.org/

University of Minnesota's page on reflexology:
www.takingcharge.csh.umn.edu/explore-healing-practices/
reflexology

Where to Buy

Juicers

Cuisinart® Pulp Control Citrus Juicer - *$29.99*

www.bedbathandbeyond.com

Hamilton Beach Big Mouth Juice Extractor - Black (Large) - *$45.99*

www.target.com

The Bistro - *£52.90*

www.bodum.co.uk

Cuisinart - *£150*

www.houseoffraser.co.uk

Kenwood - *£29.97*

www.tesco.com

Cook's Essentials - *£54.72*

www.qvcuk.com

Supplements and dietary help

Alkaline Water Jugs

biocera.com

5-day Raw Alkaline Diet Detox - recipes and videos:

http://www.alkaline-diet-health-tips.com

Royal Jelly

www.beealive.com

FertiliGreens

www.naturalfertilityshop.com

Maca Powder (US)

www.naturalfertilityshop.com

Maca Powder (UK)

www.healthysupplies.co.uk

www.hollandandbarrett.com

Fish Oils

www.nordicnaturals.com

Pure Synergy (US)   www.thesynergycompany.com
                            www.mynaturalmarket.com

Pure Synergy (UK)   www.revital.co.uk
                            www.superfooduk.com

The Organic Fertility Bible   http://www.organicfertilitybible.com

Studies

Altieri A, F. S. (2003). Epidemiology and aetiology of gestational trophoblastic diseases. *Lancet Oncol*, 670-678.

Bagshawe KD, R. G. (1971). ABO blood-groups in trophoblastic neoplasia. *Lancet*, 553-556.

Berkowitz RS, C. D. (1985). Risk factors for complete molar pregnancy from a case-control study. *Am J Obstet Gynecol*, 1016-1020.

Brinton LA, W. B. (1989). Gestatioal trophoblasic disease: a case-control study from the People's Republic of China. *Am J. Obstet Gynecol*, 121-127.

Burd, I. (2013, September). *Ectopic Pregnancy*. Retrieved December 18, 2013, from University of Maryland Medical Health Center: http://umm.edu/health/medical/pregnancy/staying-healthy-during-pregnancy/ectopic-pregnancy

Cavaliere A, E. S. (2012). Management of molar pregnancy. *J Prenat Med*, 171-175.

Diego MA, F. T.-R. (2004). Massage therapy of moderate and light pressure and vibrator effects on EEG and heart rate. *International Journal of Neuroscience*, 31-44.

Fejzo M, P. B. (2009, December). Symptoms and Pregnancy Outcomes Associated with Extreme Weight

Loss Among Women with Hyperemesis Gravidarum. *Journal of Women's Health.*

Garner EI, Lipson E, Bernstein MR, Goldstein DP, Berkowitz RS. Subsequent pregnancy experience in patients with molar pregnancy and gestational trophoblastic tumor. *J. Reprod. Med.* 47, 380–386 (2002).

Gestational Trophoblastic Disease (GTD). (2007, November 26). Retrieved December 19, 2013, from University of Michigan Health System: http://www.obgyn.med.umich.edu/sites/obgyn.med.umich.edu/files/handouts/ph_molar.pdf

Gynecologists Investigate Massage as Infertility Treatment . (2000, March 23). Retrieved December 20, 2013, from Personal MD: http://www.personalmd.com/news/n0323123924.shtml

Helwani MN, S. M. (1999). "A familial case of recurrent hydatidiform molar pregnancies with biparental genomic contribution". *Hum Genet* , 112.

Hernandez, E. (n.d.). *Gestational Trophoblastic Neoplasia.* Retrieved December 19, 2013, from Medscape: http://emedicine.medscape.com/article/279116-overview#aw2aab6b2b3

Hizli D, K. Z. (2012). Hyperemesis gravidarum and depression in pregnancy: is there an association? *Journal of Psychosomatic Obstetric & Gynecology* , 171-175.

Kohorn EI. The new FIGO 2000 staging and risk factor scoring system for gestational trophoblastic disease: description and critical assessment. *Int. J. Gynecol. Cancer* 11, 73–77 (2001).

La Vecchia C, F. S. (1985). Risk factors for gestational trophoblastic disease in Italy. *Am J Epidemiol*, 457-464.

Lorigan PC, S. S. (2000). "Characteristics of women with recurrent molar pregnancies". *Gynecol Obstet Invest*, 288-292.

Matsui H, I. Y. (2001). "Subsequent pregnancy outcome in patients with spontaneous resolution of HCG after evacuation of hydatidiform mole: comparison between complete and partial mole". *Oxford Journals*, 1274-1277.

Neimark, Jill. "The Dirty Truth About Plastic" Discover. April 18, 2008. (December 30, 2013) http://discovermagazine.com/2008/may/18-the-dirty-truth-about-plastic/?searchterm=bpa

Ozalp S, Y. O. (2001). "Recurrent molar pregnancy: report of a case with seven consecutive hydatidiform moles". *Gynecol Obstet Invest*, 215-216.

Palmer J, D. S. (1999). "Oral Contraceptive use and risks of gestational trophoblastic tumors". *JNCI Natl. Cancer Institute*, 635-640.

Schmid P, Nagai Y, Agarwal R *et al.* Prognostic markers and long-term outcome of placental-site trophoblastic tumours: a retrospective observational study. *Lancet* 374, 48–55 (2009).

Sebire NJ, F. M. (2002). "Outcome of twin pregnancies with complete hydatidiform mole and healthy co-twin". *Lancet*, 2165-2166.

Jeffrey L. Stern, M. (2007). *Trophoblastic Disease* . Retrieved December 20, 2013, from Women's Cancer Center: http://www.womenscancercenter.com/info/types/mole.html

Veenendaal MV, v. A. (2011). Consequences of hyperemesis gravidarum for offspring: a systematic review and meta-analysis. *BJOG* , 1302-2013.

Index

cysts, 11, 24, 29, 33, 43, 44, 52, 64, 105, 129

D&C, 37, 38, 40, 42, 50, 80-84, 86, 88, 121, 127

depression, 30, 31, 68, 69, 74, 76, 77, 78, 81, 82, 141

detox, 102, 103

ectopic pregnancy, 15, 16, 17, 127, 140

endometriosis, 17, 97, 102, 127

epithelioid trophoblastic tumors, 46, 51, 64, 127

exhaustion, 60, 80, 84

fallopian tube, 10, 15, 16, 17, 33, 103, 105, 110, 127, 129

folic acid, 62, 93, 96, 112, 113, 115

gestational trophoblastic neoplasia, 43, 44, 45, 126, 128

grief, 68, 69, 70, 76-79, 87, 132

GTN. See gestational trophoblastic neoplasia

hydatidiform moles, 8, 10, 11, 46, 50, 51, 63, 128

hyperemesis, 26, 29, 30, 31, 132, 141, 143

hyperthyroidism, 27, 34, 101, 102

hypothyroidism. See hyperthyroidism

hysterectomy, 39, 42, 49, 51, 55, 63-66, 75, 78, 80-85

in vitro fertilization, 17, 23, 24, 102

intercourse. See sexual intercourse

invasive mole, 10, 43, 46, 50

IVF. See in vitro fertilization

juicing, 99

liver scan tests, 54

lumbar puncture tests, 53

massage, 91, 105, 116, 140, 141

meditating, 82, 104, 105, 107, 116

meditation. See meditation

metastasize, 48, 50, 51, 53, 54, 126

metastasizing. See metastasize

methotrexate, 62, 63, 84

online forum support, 66, 69, 78, 89, 90, 132

DISCARD

CPSIA information can be obtained
at www.ICGtesting.com
Printed in the USA
LVOW04s2010211016

509751LV00008B/851/P